A SHORT COURSE
IN
EPIDEMIOLOGY

A SHORT COURSE IN EPIDEMIOLOGY

Staffan E. Norell, M.D., Ph.D.

Karolinska Institutet
Stockholm, Sweden

Raven Press ☙ New York

Raven Press, Ltd., 1185 Avenue of the Americas, New York, New York 10036

Made in the United States of America

Library of Congress Cataloging-in-Publication Data

Norell, Staffan E.
    A short course in epidemiology / Staffan E. Norell.
        p. cm.
    Includes bibliographical references and index.
    ISBN 0-88167-842-2
    1. Epidemiology. I. Title.
    [DNLM: 1. Case-Control Studies. 2. Cohort Studies. 3. Research
Design. WA 950 N834s]
    RA651.N67 1991
    614.4—dc20
    DNLM/DLC
    for Library of Congress   91-26460
                                                                    CIP

9 8 7 6 5 4 3 2 1

Preface

More and more research reports are concluding that lifestyle and environmental factors are important determinants of disease occurrence. In this context, epidemiology —the study of disease occurrence, and its relation to individual and environmental factors—is a useful tool to those wishing to understand the causes of disease. However, epidemiologic investigations are useful only to the extent that their results are accurate. Knowledge of basic research principles and of sources of error in epidemiologic studies is essential not only to those engaged in research but also to those reading research reports and evaluating the results from such studies.

This book is intended for medical students, physicians, and other health professionals with an interest in basic epidemiology. Its focus is on the design and accuracy of epidemiologic investigations. The first section of the book, Chapters 1–5, addresses cohort studies, the simplest and most straightforward design. The different sources of error, and strategies for improving validity and efficiency are discussed. These principles also apply to case-control studies as discussed in the second section, Chapters 6–10. Again, emphasis is on validity and efficiency as well as on the relation to the basic cohort design. The third section of the book, Chapters 11 and 12, addresses the choice of study design, including experimental and cross-sectional study designs, and the interpretation of results from epidemiologic investigations. Finally, tables that quantify requirements and the effects of nondifferential misclassification are provided, as is a glossary of useful epidemiologic terms.

No one can master epidemiology simply by reading about methods. Since practice is an important part of learning (and most of the fun), two chapters are devoted to exercises, many of which are based on recent papers in medical journals. Answers to the exercises are found in a separate section at the end of the book. In addition, examples are included throughout the book. The ultimate exercise still remains the critical evaluation of new epidemiologic investigations.

Staffan E. Norell, M.D., Ph.D.

Acknowledgments

I am indebted to several of my colleagues and collaborators for suggestions and support: Anders Ahlbom for stimulating discussions; Lars Alfredsson, Maria Gerhardsson, Niklas Hammar, Göran Pershagen, Gunnar Persson, Ylva Rodvall, and Denny Vàgerö for reading the manuscript; Jennifer and Walstan Wheeler for translating the text into English; and Jennifer Wheeler for typing several versions of the manuscript.

A SHORT COURSE IN EPIDEMIOLOGY

1

Introduction

Epidemiology is the study of disease occurrence and includes the study of associations between disease and characteristics of individuals and their environments. The aim is to investigate how such characteristics, or *exposures,* influence the risk of developing (or dying from) different diseases. In epidemiologic studies the occurrence of disease among exposed is compared to the occurrence among unexposed, with other factors that may influence the comparison taken into account.

Incidence is the occurrence of new cases of a disease. *Prevalence* is the proportion of subjects who have the disease at a certain point in time. The prevalence depends not only on the incidence of the disease, but also on its duration. Studies of the association between exposure and onset of disease primarily focus on disease incidence.

A difference in disease incidence between the exposed and the unexposed may be due to an effect of the exposure under study or to differences between the exposed and unexposed with respect to other factors that influence the disease incidence. Thus, the association between exposure and disease is influenced by such factors, called *confounders.* The effect of confounders is called *confounding.*

ASSOCIATION

Before an investigation, the association(s) at issue should be specified in different respects. The particular exposure and disease of interest should be defined, often both theoretically and empirically, with available examination methods borne in mind. For example, passive smoking may be defined as the "inhalation of tobacco smoke from other people's smoking," and myocardial infarction may be defined as the "necrosis (death) of heart muscle tissue" (theoretical definitions). In an empirical investigation, however, one may want to define passive smoking on the basis of the time spent with people smoking, and myocardial infarction on the basis of certain clinical or histopathological criteria. Two or more exposure categories, e.g. "exposed" and "unexposed," are defined on the basis of the amount of exposure that could be expected to influence the occurrence of disease. Several aspects may be taken into account, such as the intensity, duration, and frequency of exposure. In addition, the risk of myocardial infarction, for example, may be affected only several years after the exposure occurred. Thus, specifications should also be made as to the expected time relation between exposure and effect, the *induction time*. Finally, the question may be whether the incidence is higher (and if so, how much higher) among exposed than among unexposed, with other factors (confounders) that could influence the comparison—for example, smoking, blood pressure, and previous heart disease in the case of myocardial infarction—taken into account. For every association between exposure and disease that is studied, a decision should be made in terms of the following:

1. What disease is to be studied? [Definition: (a) theoretical, (b) empirical on the basis of diagnostic criteria and examination methods used.]
2. What exposure is to be studied? [Definition: (a) theoretical, (b) empirical on the basis of criteria and examination methods used.]
3. What is the induction time, that is, the time relation between exposure and effect (occurrence of the disease)?
4. What are the relevant confounders? [Definition: (a) theoretical, (b) empirical on the basis of criteria and examination methods used.]

Exposure may influence the disease occurrence differently among different sections of the population; this is called *effect modification.* The association should therefore be specified in yet another respect: In what section of the population is the association to be studied? An example of such specification is "the effect of a high intake of polyunsaturated fats on the risk of breast cancer in premenopausal women," if the effect among such women can differ from the corresponding effect among older women (and among men). If one wants to study the effect of the exposure in different sections of the population, the various segments must be adequately represented in the investigation. Otherwise the question (and the investigation) should be limited to a particular section of the population. If, for example, the great majority of the available subjects with a certain occupational exposure are men, perhaps the questions and the investigation should be limited to apply to men, if the exposure may have different effects between men and women. Effect modification is also involved in conjunction with the question of the generalizability of the results. The question of the conditions under which an observed association can be considered to represent a causal association is discussed in Chapter 12.

STUDY BASE

The association between exposure and disease is studied in a sample of the population in question, e.g. a sample of premenopausal women. This sample, the *study population*, is observed with respect to onset of the disease during a defined period of time, the *follow-up period.*

The study population should be defined at the start of the follow-up period. Since the follow-up period is used to observe for onset of disease, all individuals must be free of the studied disease at the start of the follow-up period—and prior to this, if the study concerns onset of disease for the first time. The study population may be: (1) a *closed population,* which means that the same individuals are followed from the start of the follow-up period until its end (or until their deaths), or (2) an *open population,* into or out of which individuals move during the follow-up period, e.g., the population in a town, with people moving in and out. Open and closed populations differ in several respects; for example, individuals in a closed population, but not necessarily an open one, grow older as time passes.

The follow-up period is usually defined in calendar time, for example, "January 1–December 31, 1992." In certain situations the follow-up period is defined otherwise, e.g., "during the first year of life" (a period that may vary in calendar time depending on the date of birth). One consequence of this is that "children born in Boston during the period January 1, 1990–December 31, 1992 and followed during their first year of life" are to be regarded as a closed population where the follow-up period is one year (varying in calendar time).

The *study base* (Fig. 1.1) is the "person-time-experience" studied with regard to disease occurrence, i.e., the study population during the follow-up period (Miettinen 1982b). This is the "base" of the study insofar as it is the person-time in which the effect of the exposure is studied. Its size depends on the size of the study population and the length of the follow-up period. In addition, one should take into account any mortality during the follow-up period—and individuals developing the studied disease, if the incidence is high (otherwise this is negligible). If the study population is an open one, account must be taken of the fact that individuals move in or out of the study during the follow-up period.

STUDY DESIGN

The principles of study design are based on an overall goal: to obtain accurate results with limited resources. *Accuracy* is the extent to which the result reflects the effect of the exposure on the risk of developing the disease (in the study base). Accuracy depends on *validity,* i.e., the absence of *systematic*

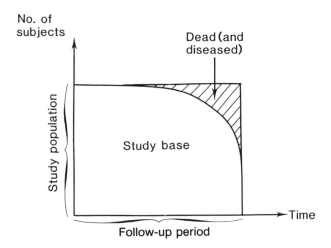

FIG. 1.1. The study base is the "person-time-experience" studied with regard to disease occurrence. Here the study population is a closed one.

errors such as confounding and misclassification with respect to exposure and disease, respectively. In addition, accuracy depends on *precision,* i.e., the absence of *random errors* that occur when results are based on small numbers. Precision can be improved by increasing the size of the study, but usually this also increases the costs. There are different ways to improve the relation between precision and cost, i.e., the *efficiency* (or cost-efficiency) of a study.

Epidemiologic studies aimed at investigating the association between exposure and onset of disease (with information on an individual basis) are usually divided into cohort studies and case-control studies (e.g., MacMahon, Pugh 1970). Cohort studies (Chapter 2) are based on exposure information from the whole study base. This information is usually collected prior to follow-up. The exposed and unexposed are compared with regard to occurrence of disease during the follow-up period. Cohort studies are based, as a rule, on closed populations. The term *cohort study* or *follow-up study* is sometimes used only for such studies based on closed populations.

However, similar studies may, in principle, also be based on open populations. In cohort studies, systematic errors (Chapter 3) may occur if the exposed and unexposed differ in terms of other factors that affect the occurrence of disease (confounding), or if the methods used for examination and classification with regard to exposure and disease, respectively, are not accurate (misclassification). Most diseases have low or moderate incidence; thus, a very large number of individuals must be examined for the study to embrace a sufficient number of cases of the disease. Precision and efficiency (Chapter 4) are therefore often important problems in cohort studies.

Case-control studies (Chapter 6) are based on exposure information from the cases and a sample of the study base (Miettinen 1985a). The aim is improved efficiency relative to the corresponding cohort study. Case-control studies may be designed in different ways (Chapters 7–9) and are often, but not always, based on open populations. As in the corresponding cohort study, systematic errors may occur because of confounding or misclassification. In some case-control studies special problems may occur with regard to exposure misclassification (Chapter 8) and the sampling of the study base [the selection of so-called controls (Chapter 9)]. The choice between a cohort or a case-control design is based on consideration of these problems, as well as of efficiency, for the particular association (exposure and disease) to be studied.

The choice of study design (Chapter 11) is not limited to cohort and case-control strategies but includes experimental, cross-sectional, and other designs. In the interpretation of results (Chapter 12), there are two basic questions: Does the result reflect the effect of the exposure in the study base (accuracy)? If so, to what extent does the result apply outside the study base (generalizability)?

2

Cohort Design

A *cohort study* (follow-up study) is an investigation of the association between exposure and the onset of disease in which use is made of exposure information from the whole study base.

In cohort studies an estimation and comparison is made of the disease incidence between the exposed and unexposed. The aim is to analyze any association between exposure and disease. The groups may differ, however, in other respects—for example, in terms of age and sex distribution or the occurrence of other relevant exposure—and this may affect the result of the comparison. One way of handling this problem is to assign exposure at random. Experimental studies (see, for example, Chapter 11) may be described as a special variant of cohort studies. For ethical reasons, the intervention is usually an attempt to reduce the frequency of an exposure that is assumed to increase the disease incidence. Major practical problems are often met here. Strict randomization at the individual level may, for example, be difficult or impossible to carry out. Perhaps the most serious limitation, however, as far as the use of randomized experiments in epidemiology is concerned, is not the ethical and practical problems but the fact that such a design is often inefficient for studying the association between exposure and disease (Chapter 11). Despite these limitations, it may be suitable in certain situations to design epidemiologic studies as randomized experiments.

In cohort studies, as in other epidemiologic studies of the association between exposure and disease, it is often suitable to use existing exposure conditions as the point of departure. It is sometimes said that the accuracy of such a cohort study depends on exposed and unexposed individuals being similar in all respects, except in terms of the studied exposure. This is a misconception. In the first place, the comparison is affected only by differences with respect to factors that influence the incidence of the disease being studied. Second, the effect of such factors (confounding) may be prevented in the selection of the study base or suitably controlled in the data analysis. This is, however, one of the most important questions in epidemiologic methodology and is discussed in greater detail in Chapter 3.

PRINCIPLES OF COHORT DESIGN

The principles of a cohort study may be described according to Fig. 2.1. The study base is the person-time observed with respect to disease occurrence, i.e., the study population during the follow-up period (Chapter 1). The study population—which, as a rule, is a closed population—is examined with regard to exposure conditions (including potential confounders) and observed during the follow-up period with regard to occurrence of the disease studied.

Regarding disease occurrence, the investigation is often restricted to apply to the first onset of the disease (or possibly development of the disease for the second time, for example, the risk to individuals who have had one myocardial infarction of developing a second infarction). The number of individuals that develop the disease is then the same as the number of cases of the disease studied. In certain situations, however, the investigation includes repeated onsets of the disease, in which case one individual may contribute several cases of the studied disease. In that event, account must be taken of the fact that the risk of falling sick may be influenced

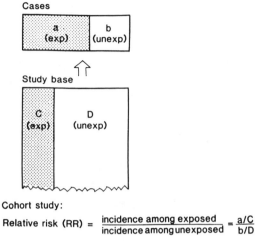

Cohort study:

Relative risk (RR) = $\dfrac{\text{incidence among exposed}}{\text{incidence among unexposed}}$ = $\dfrac{a/C}{b/D}$

FIG. 2.1 Principles of cohort design.

by whether or not a subject had the disease earlier; the risk of developing a myocardial infarction, for example, increases if a person has had an infarction previously, whereas the risk of contracting certain infectious diseases diminishes if a person has already had the disease and as a result has acquired a specific immunity.

In the study, a comparison is made between the incidence of the disease in the exposed (a/C) and unexposed (b/D), (see Fig. 2.1). The *relative risk* (or *rate ratio*) is the disease incidence in the exposed divided by the incidence in the unexposed. There may also be an interest in the *rate difference,* i.e., the difference in incidence between the exposed and the unexposed. The comparison is often based on *incidence rate,* where a and b in Fig. 2.1 are the number of cases among the exposed and unexposed, respectively, and C and D are the number of person-years among the exposed and unexposed, respectively, in the study base.

In certain situations, the comparison is based on *cumulative incidence,* where a and b represent the number of individuals developing the disease among the exposed and unexposed, respectively, and C and D represent the number of exposed and unexposed individuals, respectively, at the commence-ment of the follow-up period. Hence, when comparisons are based on cumulative incidence, the study base is replaced by the study population. In a comparison of this kind, account is not taken of any differences in mortality between exposed and unexposed individuals. If the mortality is higher among exposed than among unexposed individuals, this results in an underestimation of the relative risk. If the incidence of the studied disease is high, any differences in incidence between the exposed and unexposed may influence the comparison correspondingly. When the study population is an open one, the comparison cannot be based on cumulative incidence since individuals move in and out of the study population during the follow-up period.

Investigations of the association between exposure and onset of disease should, in principle, be based on comparisons of incidence. In certain situations—for example, those involving congenital malformations—only information about prevalent cases is available. Investigations based on the comparison of prevalence (cross-sectional studies) are dis-cussed in Chapter 11.

A cohort study is essentially conducted in three stages: (1) choice of study base, (2) examination and classification with respect to exposure (including potential confounders), and (3) follow-up and classification regarding onset of disease.

CHOICE OF STUDY BASE

The choice of study base (i.e., study population and follow-up period) is important to the validity and efficiency of the investigation (Chapters 3–4). A common misconception is that the individuals selected for the investigation should be representative of the "whole population" (Chapter 12). Instead, individuals should be selected with regard to the validity and efficiency of the investigation. This may mean, for example, that the selection should be limited to middle-aged men, to women who work in certain occupations, or to people who are not smokers.

In the selection of the study base, the conditions that should be taken into account include the following (for details and examples, see Chapters 3 and 4):

1. Regarding the studied disease:
   a. The incidence of the disease and the strength of the association in the study base (Chapter 4).
   b. The possibilities of identifying all cases that occur in the study base (Chapter 3).
2. Regarding the studied exposure:
   a. The occurrence of the exposure in the study base (Chapter 4).
   b. The possibilities of establishing exposure in the study base (Chapter 3).
3. Regarding relevant confounders:
   a. The occurrence of confounders in the study base (Chapter 3).
   b. The possibilities of establishing confounders in the study base.

The efficiency of the investigation is influenced by the disease incidence and the strength of the association (1a) and by the occurrence of the exposure (2a) in the study base. The validity is influenced by the basis for classification with respect to the disease (1b) and exposure (2b), as well as by the possibilities of avoiding or controlling or confounding (3). The choice of study base is consequently important for the avoidance of both systematic errors (confounding, misclassification) and random errors.

The size of the study base should be chosen with due regard to the precision of the investigation (Chapter 4). This is often a problem in cohort studies of diseases with a low or moderate incidence, which require examination of exposure conditions in a very large number of individuals to ensure adequate precision. The use of register data may, in certain situations, provide large study bases suitable for cohort studies.

CLASSIFICATION

The subjects included in the study population are examined and classified with respect to exposure conditions and disease onset during the follow-up period.

Exposure

All individuals are examined and classified with regard to exposure conditions, including potential confounders. [What is to be considered an exposure or a potential confounder depends on the association being studied (Chapter 3)]. Various methods may be used, but as a rule the process embraces the following stages: (1) definition of specific exposure, (2) decision regarding the induction period, (3) choice of method of examination, and (4) subdivision into different exposure categories. Misclassification with respect to exposure is discussed in Chapter 3.

Definition

The exposure may be defined theoretically on the basis of the etiological question and empirically on the basis of the examination methods used in the study. Suppose, for example, that one wants to investigate how exposure to X-rays influences the risk of developing breast cancer. Theoretically, exposure may be defined and quantified on the basis of the amount of X-rays that strike the breast tissues. However, bearing in mind the criteria and the examination methods to be used in a particular study, one might want to define exposure empirically on the basis of the number of X-ray examinations in which the breast is exposed (e.g., chest X-rays). Differences between the theoretical and empirical definitions of exposure may result in misclassification. Most exposures may be considered continuous variables. Attention should be paid to several aspects, including the type, quantity, frequency, duration, and timing of exposure.

Example 2.1: An investigation has been planned to study the association between smoking and certain respiratory cancers. Exposure can be divided into smoking of cigarettes, cigarillos, cigars, and pipes. Cigarette smoking may be quantified on the basis of the number of cigarettes smoked per day. There may, however, also be reason to pay attention to the duration of smoking, age at which subject started smoking, type of cigarettes smoked (tar content, filter, etc.), and manner of smoking (inhaling, length of stub, etc.). The theoretical starting point is the inhaled amount of certain chemical components of tobacco smoke. The aspects that should be taken into account regarding smoking habits naturally depend on what may be expected to influence this exposure, and consequently the danger of falling sick, and on the possibilities (and the cost) related to the examination of the exposure conditions.

Induction Period

Classification with respect to exposure presupposes a decision on the time relation between the exposure and effect (onset of disease)—the induction period. This varies for different exposure-disease associations (from hours or days for certain bacteria/infectious diseases to one or more decades for certain carcinogens/malignant tumor diseases). If, for example, the induction time is 10 years and the follow-up period is 5 years, information about exposure conditions should be collected 5 to 10 years before the start of the follow-up period. If the interview or questionnaire methodology is used, questions about exposure conditions 5 to 10 years earlier may be asked at the beginning of the follow-up period (retrospective exposure information). If the induction time is unknown and exposure conditions show considerable variations in time, exposure data should be collected in such a way that classification may be made with varying assumptions regarding the length of the induction period.

Example 2.2: To take into account different induction times ("tumor initiation" and/or "promotion") in Example 2.1, the exposure may be divided into different time periods (for example, 5- or 10-year periods) before the follow-up period.

Method of Examination

Procedures for the collection of data may vary from chemical and physical methods of measurement to interview or questionnaire methodology. For many exposures it may be possible to use well-established examination methods along with special competence in the current sector. However, the choice of examination method presupposes familiarity with epidemiologic methodology. The effect of a particular misclassification in a cohort study (or case-control study), for example, differs considerably from the effect of a corresponding misclassification in an investigation aimed at describing the occurrence of the exposure (see, for example, Chapter 5, Exercise 2). The effect of any misclassification must also be weighed against the random errors introduced if fewer individuals can be studied using an expensive method and the systematic errors that may be introduced if the participation rate decreases with a complicated method (Chapters 3 and 4).

Example 2.3: In the investigation of smoking and cancer morbidity (Example 2.1), standardized interviews were carried out immediately before the start of the follow-up period regarding smoking habits (and potential confounders) according to a questionnaire with encoded, fixed answer alternatives. Exposure conditions included current smoking habits as well as smoking habits 5, 10, 15, and 20 years earlier. The questions referred to the number (and type) of cigarettes, cigarillos, and cigars smoked per day and the number of grams of pipe tobacco smoked per week. Questions were also asked about the manner of smoking (inhaling, etc.) and the year the subject started/gave up smoking.

A small-scale investigation might include a discussion of the possibilities of using a completely different examination method, for example, the analysis of cotinine in urine (an excretion product of nicotine) as a measure of the current exposure to tobacco smoke. In choosing the examination method, however, primary attention should be paid not to the method that best reflects the theoretically defined exposure, but to the way in which the results of the investigation are influenced by differences related to misclassification, nonparticipation, and cost (study size).

Subdivision

The range of conceivable examination results should be subdivided into mutually exclusive categories. In determining subdivisions, attention should naturally be paid to the levels at which exposure may be expected to influence morbidity. A subdivision is usually made into three (or more) categories: exposed, unexposed, and others. The "others" include individuals who could not be examined or for whom the examination results do not permit a classification as exposed or unexposed. It may be useful to subdivide the exposed into two or more categories, for example, low exposed and high exposed. Every exposure level is then compared with the unexposed with regard to disease incidence. When a large number of categories is used, precision diminishes because of the limited number of cases of the disease at every exposure level (Chapter 4).

Example 2.4: In the investigation described (in Example 2.1) results were first divided into the following exposure categories: (1) cigarettes: ≥ 25 per day, 15–24 per day, ≤ 14 per day; (2) pipe and/or cigars/cigarillos; and (3) combination of cigarettes and cigarillos, cigars, and/or pipe. The subdivision was made for different time periods corresponding to differing assumptions regarding the length of the induction time. For every period comparison was made of every category of exposed with the unexposed (those who had never smoked). The effects of age of commencement and manner of smoking were studied separately.

Disease

The aim is to identify all new cases of the studied disease occurring in the study base. Exposure must not influence the identification of the cases. Misclassification in relation to disease is discussed in Chapter 3.

A decision should be reached regarding diagnostic criteria and examination methods. The principles for examination and classification with respect to disease are described elsewhere (see, for example, Ahlbom, Norell 1990, Chapter 3). In certain situations exposure may affect the diagnostics of the disease, and this may introduce a systematic error in the investigation. To avoid this, follow-up and examination routines should be identical for exposed and unexposed individuals. This may mean that criteria and examination methods used as a matter of routine must be changed; for example, the diagnosis may be made "blind" (without knowledge of the exposure conditions).

Example 2.5: In planning an investigation of the association between smoking and chronic bronchitis, it turned out that doctors were more inclined to diagnose chronic bronchitis if they knew that the patient was a smoker. This would introduce a systematic error in the investigation and result in an overestimation of the relative risk. To avoid this, the possibility was discussed of conducting the examination and diagnosis blind, that is, without knowledge of the patient's smoking habits.

In identifying the cases it is essential to distinguish between occurrence of disease and utilization of medical services. For many diseases, only a limited proportion of the cases lead to a visit to the doctor or contact with medical services. If the proportion differs among exposed and unexposed people, a systematic error is introduced when only those cases that have received medical services are identified. To avoid this, the follow-up should be so designed that all cases of the disease occurring are identified, irrespective of contact with medical services. This may create considerable practical problems, especially for diseases with a low incidence and short duration, where only a small or moderate proportion of the persons developing the disease normally visit a doctor. For a disease where almost 100 percent of the people who develop it visit a doctor (or die) and the disease is diagnosed, this is a considerably smaller problem. Even with such diseases, however, every case may lead to one or more medical visits or hospitalizations, and it is disease occurrence rather than medical care consumption that is to be studied.

Example 2.6: Chronic bronchitis is a disease that does not always lead to a visit to the doctor. If smokers are more inclined to visit the doctor when suffering from a complaint of the respiratory tract than nonsmokers, this would introduce a systematic error in the investigation and result in an overestimation of the relative risk. To avoid this, the investigators discussed the possibility of basing the follow-up of disease occurrence on some form of visiting activity.

Example 2.7: Hip fractures almost always lead to hospitalization. Therefore, in an investigation of the association between certain environmental factors and hip fracture, it was decided to use a hospitalization register for the follow-up of disease occurrence. Sometimes, however, two or more instances of hospitalization turned out to involve the same disease case. Furthermore, several elderly patients suffered hip fractures during hospitalization on account of another disease. The follow-up period refers to the time of the onset of the disease, not to the time of discharge from the hospital or entry in the hospitalization register. This must be taken into account in a follow-up with regard to the occurrence of disease.

Sometimes the yield of a cohort study can be increased by carrying out the follow-up with regard to more than one disease that is of interest in relation to the studied exposure conditions.

3

Systematic Error

With regard to the accuracy of the results, it is usual to distinguish systematic error (i.e., bias) and random error (see Chapter 4). *Systematic errors* are those that would give an average deviation from the true value if the investigation were repeated an infinite number of times with the same methodology. (An analogy is the pattern of hits from a rifle with an incorrectly adjusted sight.) Systematic errors may result in an underestimation of the relative risk ($RR \rightarrow 0$), an overestimation of the relative risk ($RR \rightarrow \infty$), or a "diluting effect," i.e., an underestimation of the strength of the association ($RR \rightarrow 1$). *Validity* is the absence of systematic errors.

Systematic errors may occur if the exposed and unexposed differ with regard to other factors that affect the risk of developing the disease (confounding) or if the information pertaining to exposure or disease is erroneous (misclassification). Systematic errors may be avoided or controlled at different stages of an investigation—confounding in the choice of study base, in data analysis, and through randomization in experimental studies; misclassification in the examination with respect to exposure and disease and, to a certain extent, also in the choice of study base and during data analysis. Subdivision of systematic errors is discussed in brief at the end of this chapter.

CONFOUNDING

When the exposed and unexposed differ with regard to the occurrence of other factors that influence the risk of falling ill, this may introduce a systematic error into the investigation. A factor that influences the comparability between the exposed and unexposed in this way is called a *confounder* (or a *confounding factor*), and the systematic error that it introduces is called *confounding*. What should be considered an exposure or a confounder depends on the association being studied. Assume, for example, that there is a covariance between smoking and alcohol consumption, and that both smoking and alcohol consumption influence the risk of developing cancer of the throat. Smoking is then a confounder when the association between alcohol consumption and cancer of the throat is studied. Alcohol consumption is a confounder when—perhaps within the framework of the same investigation—the association between smoking and cancer of the throat is studied. Defined formally, then, a *confounder* is a factor that (1) is covariant with the studied exposure in the study base and (2) influences the risk of developing the studied disease (over and above what is occasioned by any association between exposure and disease). Figure 3.1 illustrates confounding in diagram form.

Covariance with the studied exposure in the study base may arise in different ways. One possibility is that the study base was chosen from a population in which the confounding

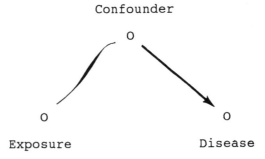

FIG. 3.1. Diagrammatic illustration of confounding.

factor is covariant with the exposure, for example, one in which smokers have a greater tendency to drink alcohol than nonsmokers. Another possibility is that the study base was selected in such a way as to include a covariance that does not occur in the general population. If, on the other hand, the selection for an investigation of the association between smoking and cancer of the throat was made in such a way that smoking and alcohol are not covariant in the study base, alcohol is not a confounder in the investigation, even if there is a covariance between smoking and alcohol consumption in the general population. The decisive factor is thus whether there is covariance with the studied exposure in the study base, irrespective of how this covariance arose. However, it is not sufficient that there is covariance among the cases, which may be a consequence of both the exposure and factor in question influencing the risk of onset of disease.

A confounder also influences the risk of developing the studied disease. Theoretically, this means that the factor in question should be a (contributing) cause of the disease. Like exposure, a confounder may be defined empirically as well as theoretically. In an investigation of the association between exposure to sunlight and cancer of the skin, for example, pigmentation is a potential confounder, but in practice one must often be content with such known and measurable indicators as eye or hair color. In addition, many specific causes of disease are unknown, and their effects on the comparability between exposed and unexposed can only be controlled via other risk indicators (e.g., age, sex, place of residence, socioeconomic group). In practice, therefore, the condition that the factor in question influences the risk of developing the studied disease means that it should be a risk indicator for the disease.

A confounder is a risk indicator for the studied disease beyond what is occasioned by any association between exposure and disease. If, for example, lung cancer is more common among individuals who drink alcohol, alcohol consumption is a risk indicator for lung cancer. In an investigation of the association between smoking and lung cancer, however, alcohol is not a confounder if the association between alcohol and lung cancer is only a consequence of the covariance between smoking and alcohol consumption. This situation is illustrated in Fig. 3.2a, in which X (alcohol consumption) is not a confounder.

The fact that a confounder is a risk indicator over and above what is brought on by any association between exposure and disease means that exposure and confounder are linked to different causal chains. If, for example, exposure to certain infectious agents gives rise to tonsillitis and this in its turn gives rise to arthritis, then tonsillitis is not a confounder in an investigation of the association between exposure to infectious agents and arthritis. This situation is illustrated in Fig 3.2b, where X (tonsillitis) is not a confounder.

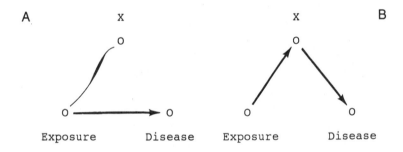

FIG. 3.2. A, B: Two situations where X is *not* a confounder.

As mentioned earlier, the association between confounder and disease is based on the etiology of the disease. It has therefore been suggested that an a priori decision should be taken regarding the factors that are known risk indicators for the studied disease (Miettinen, Cook 1981). In practice, however, many risk indicators are unknown and may be identified for the first time in the current investigation. In view of this, it may be justifiable to reach a decision on the basis of the results: A confounder will arise as a risk indicator for the disease both among the exposed and the unexposed. The effect of a potential confounder may be studied by means of stratification in data analysis.

A confounder may be positively or negatively covariant

with the exposure, and indicate an increased or decreased risk of disease. Confounding may therefore result in over- or underestimation of the relative risk. For a confounder to account for an appreciable over- or underestimation of the relative risk however, it must have a strong covariance with the exposure, and its association with the disease must be stronger than that observed for the exposure. The systematic error introduced by a confounder concerns the association between a certain exposure and a certain disease in a certain study base. The effect is dependent, however, on the other confounders that are taken into account in the analysis.

Example 3.1: In an investigation of the association between stress and mortality from myocardial infarction, confounders included marital status and area of residence (degree of urbanization). There was a greater proportion of single persons and a greater proportion of individuals living in an urban area among the exposed than among the unexposed. Mortality from myocardial infarction was greater among single than among married persons and greater in urban than in rural areas. In addition, there was a considerable covariance between marital status and area of residence: single persons constituted a greater proportion of the population in urban than in rural areas. Thus, the confounding effects from marital status and degree of urbanization were, to a large extent, the same effect. After confounding from degree of urbanization was controlled for, nearly the whole effect of marital status as a confounder was eliminated at the same time.

In practice, age and gender are almost always regarded as potential confounders. The confounding effect can be avoided by restricting the study base (e.g., by limiting the investigation to men) or controlled in the data analysis (e.g., by stratifying based on age). Other potential confounders that should be taken into account, such as area of residence (urbanization, region, etc.), socioeconomic group, nationality, and marital status, depend on the association (exposure and disease) being studied. The possibility of a covariance of a known risk indicator or contributing cause of the studied disease with the studied exposure should always be considered. If, for example, one wants to investigate how exposure to radon influences the risk of developing lung cancer, smoking should be taken into account as a potential confounder. For certain diseases it is easy to list a large number of known risk indicators. In practice, however, only a limited number of these will be sufficiently covariant with the studied exposure to create any appreciable confounding. In addition, these factors are often covariant with one another. Taking into account a small number of important confounders in the data analysis or restricting the study base will often reduce the remaining effect of other confounders. In general, confounders with a very uneven distribution among the exposed and/or unexposed are best dealt with by restriction in the choice of study base (e.g., to men if sex is a confounder and there are few exposed women). Stratification in the data analysis is an alternative for confounders with a more even distribution.

Certain potential confounders may be difficult to define or measure, e.g., lifestyle, general state of health, or psychosocial conditions. As a rule, exposed and unexposed subjects should be chosen so that the groups are similar in such respects. For example, if one wants to study the effect of a specific chemical exposure in a certain occupation, it would be possible to choose an unexposed group from the general population. It may, however, be better to choose an occupational group that resembles the exposed group except for the studied exposure. One reason for this is the so-called healthy worker effect (McMichael 1976), i.e., that those employed in a particular occupation may have a better general state of health and consequently a smaller risk of developing the disease compared with the rest of the population (which includes, for example, unemployed persons and those on early retirement). It may be useful to consider "exposure" as a state that individuals under certain conditions may choose (or be influenced) to enter or leave. For certain occupations (and connected exposures) a good general state of health is required; at the same time, the individuals whose health deteriorates tend to change over to less arduous work (or resort to sick leave or early retirement) and consequently cease to be exposed.

Another source of confounding is that a certain type of job or lifestyle, for example, may involve several exposures in addition to the specific one under study. This problem may be avoided by selecting an unexposed group that is similar to the exposed group in these respects.

Example 3.2: Conceivable associations between certain chemical exposures at work and myocardial infarction have been discussed. To study a possible association between exposure to soot and mortality from myocardial infarction, information from the Swedish census of 1960 and the Cause-of-Death Register for 1961–80 were used. Chimney sweeps and other gainfully employed men between the ages of 20 and 64 years in the census of 1960 were followed up with the use of the Cause-of-Death Register and compared for mortality due to myocardial infarction. It is important, however, to distinguish exposure to soot from work as a chimney sweep according to the census of 1960. The reasons for this include the following (see also Example 3.4):

1. If men with a good general state of health (e.g., the absence of cardiovascular disease) are overrepresented among chimney sweeps due to demands for a good general state of health within the profession, chimney sweeps may be a sample with a lower risk of dying from myocardial infarction than other men—irrespective of any effect due to exposure. On comparison with other men in the census of 1960, this would mean an underestimation of the relative risk due to confounding from a good general state of health (healthy worker effect). The effect may diminish if the comparison group is limited to men in other occupations (with unemployed and persons on early retirement among those excluded). To avoid such confounding, it may be suitable, however, to choose the comparison group from other occupations with corresponding requirements for a good general state of health.

2. A chimney sweep's work may involve other exposure (in addition to soot) that influences the risk of myocardial infarction. If, for example, stress is more common among chimney sweeps than those in other occupations, this may lead to an overestimation of the relative risk. To avoid such confounding, it may be suitable to choose the comparison group from occupations with a corresponding amount of stress. Similarly, in

the choice of a comparison group, one may take into account confounding from, for example, socioeconomic status.

If the studied exposure influences mortality, the surviving individuals may differ from the rest in terms of the risk of developing a disease, irrespective of any effect of exposure on disease occurrence (healthy survivor effect). Assume, for example, that a certain proportion of individuals exposed to high doses of ionizing radiation die a short time after exposure, and that the survivors, irrespective of the effects of the radiation, have a good general state of health and a lower risk of developing, for example, cancer. In an investigation of the association between exposure to high doses of radiation and the risk of developing cancer, confounding from a good general state of health would consequently give an underestimation of the relative risk. It may be difficult to find an unexposed group that is comparable with the survivors among the exposed persons.

One form of confounding that deserves particular attention arises when "preliminary stages" (or previous episodes) of the studied disease influence the occurrence of exposure.

Example 3.3.: In an investigation of the association between coffee consumption and development of a stomach ulcer, the disease incidence was compared among individuals with different coffee drinking habits who, at the start of the follow-up period, were free of the studied disease. It was seen, however, that many of those who developed an ulcer during the follow-up period had had the disease earlier and subsequently had reduced their coffee consumption. It was also shown that many of those who developed an ulcer during the follow-up period, but who had not had the disease previously, had had stomach complaints (pain in the epigastrium, acid regurgitations, etc.) previously and subsequently had reduced their coffee consumption. Confounding from an earlier ulcer or stomach complaints would consequently produce a systematic error in the direction of RR=0.

This type of confounding may be difficult or impossible to control in data analysis. Sometimes the problem may be handled by restriction in choice of the study base (e.g., by including only individuals who have not had an ulcer or stomach complaints). In certain situations, however, the problem may be so difficult to handle that it is preferable to refrain from conducting the investigation.

MISCLASSIFICATION

Misclassification with respect to exposure or disease may vary in type and extent. This influences the effect on the investigation's results and the choice of measures for dealing with the problem.

Exposure

In nearly all investigations, some misclassification occurs with respect to exposure. In every investigation an appraisal should be made as to how misclassification can influence the results and as to what measures should be taken to reduce the resulting inaccuracy. These appraisals depend on the type and extent of the misclassification. It may be useful to consider three different types of misclassification:

1. *Misclassification independent of the studied disease:* The probability of misclassification in relation to exposure is similar for those who develop the disease and for those who do not—so-called nondifferential misclassification.
2. *Misclassification influenced by a risk indicator for the studied disease:* Age, for example, may influence the accuracy of certain interview or questionnaire data concerning exposure and also constitute a risk indicator for the studied disease. Misclassification of this kind is nondifferential within strata, i.e., among individuals who are similar to one another with respect to the risk indicator in question (e.g., within the framework of an age group).
3. *Misclassification influenced by the studied disease:* This does not arise in cohort studies, where the exposure information is collected before the follow-up period, but occurs in investigations where the exposure information is not

collected until after the cases have been identified (Chapters 8 and 9).

As mentioned previously, the methods of examination and classification with regard to exposure may vary considerably. The extent of the misclassification is determined by the *sensitivity* of the method (the probability that an exposed individual will be classified as exposed) and the *specificity* (the probability that an unexposed individual will be classified as unexposed). In nondifferential misclassification, sensitivity and specificity, respectively, are the same among those who develop the disease and those who do not. The same is true for the second type of misclassification, once the sample has been stratified for the risk indicator in question. The third type of misclassification has the most serious effect on the result of the investigation (Chapter 8).

Fortunately, misclassification is often independent of the studied disease. A common source of such misclassification is a "blunted" examination method, e.g., a questionnaire that does not provide sufficiently precise information about the studied exposure, resulting in some exposed individuals being misclassified as unexposed and/or vice versa. Another common source of nondifferential misclassification is exposure information that refers to the wrong time period in relation to the induction time, e.g., food habits immediately before the start of the follow-up period rather than 5 to 10 years previously. The extent of the misclassification and, consequently, the effect on the results of the investigation depend on the extent to which the exposure conditions vary over a period of time.

Nondifferential misclassification with respect to exposure results in a diluting effect, leading to an underestimation of the strength of the association, i.e., influencing the relative risk in the direction of $RR=1$ (e.g., Flegal et al. 1986). This applies regardless of whether the method gives an over- or underestimation of the occurrence of the exposure (providing, however, that the method is no worse than random procedure for distinguishing exposed and unexposed subjects). Even a considerable misclassification has a fairly moderate effect on the strength of the observed association. In Table 3.1, for example, a 50% underestimation of the number of exposed individuals would give RR=1.8 rather than the true value, RR=2.0 (see also Table 13.1). Nondifferential misclassification is not a reason for questioning results that show an association between exposure and disease, even if it may lead to an underestimation of the strength of the association. Investigation results that do not show an association may, on the other hand, be questioned on account of the misclassification possibly concealing an association. If the sensitivity and specificity of the method are known, it is possible to assess the effect of the misclassification on the result and correct this (e.g., Greenland, Kleinbaum 1983).

Example 3.4: The investigation of the association between exposure to soot and mortality from myocardial infarction was discussed in Example 3.2. Chimney sweeps were compared with men working in other occupations according to the census of 1960. Misclassification in terms of exposure may arise on account of some of the men who were working as chimney sweeps in 1960 not having been exposed to soot to any large

TABLE 3.1. Misclassification with regard to exposure (nondifferential misclassification)

	Exposed	Unexposed	Relative risk
Number of individuals	2,000	8,000	
Number of cases	20	40	2.0
Underestimation of exposure (sens. = 0.5, spec. = 1.0):			
Number of individuals identified	1,000	9,000	
Number of cases identified	10	50	1.8
Overestimation of exposure (sens. = 1.0, spec. = 0.5):			
Number of individuals identified	6,000	4,000	
Number of cases identified	40	20	1.3

Sens., sensitivity; spec., specificity.

extent (because of a short time in the profession or special working conditions) and some of the men who worked in other occupations in 1960 having been exposed to soot (in earlier work as chimney sweeps, in other occupations, or in their leisure time). Such an intermixture of unexposed individuals among "exposed" and vice versa is likely to lead to an underestimation of the strength of the association (i.e., influence the relative risk in the direction of RR=1). Misclassification with respect to exposure may also arise on account of insufficient attention being paid to the induction time. Men who were working as chimney sweeps in 1960 were observed for mortality from myocardial infarction during the period 1961–80. If the induction time is long (e.g., 10 years or more), and if a large proportion of those who were chimney sweeps in 1960 were not working in this occupation 10 years earlier, this would also result in an underestimation of the strength of the association, particularly for the earlier part of the follow-up period. It may then be suitable to make separate comparisons, for example, using the periods 1961–70 and 1971–80.

Misclassification influenced by a risk indicator for the studied disease (e.g., age) may give an over- or underestimation of the relative risk. If the risk indicator is treated as a confounder in the investigation (for example, by means of stratification in the data analysis), the effect will always be an underestimation of the strength of the association (i.e., the relative risk is influenced in the direction of RR=1). On the other hand, the relative risk after stratification is not always closer to the "true" value. (See, for example, Greenland, Robins 1985.) In certain situations, this type of misclassification may be reduced through restriction in the choice of study base, for example, by means of an upper age limit if the probability of misclassification increases with high age.

Disease

To avoid systematic errors, all cases of the disease that occur in the study base should be identified. Misclassification in terms of disease may be of different kinds:

1. *Misclassification independent of the studied exposure:* The probability of misclassification with respect to disease is the same for exposed and unexposed individuals—so-called nondifferential misclassification.
2. *Misclassification influenced by a factor that is covariant with the studied exposure:* Age for example, may be covariant with the exposure and at the same time affect accuracy as far as follow-up and diagnosis with regard to certain diseases are concerned. Such misclassification is independent within strata, i.e., among individuals who are similar in terms of the factor in question (e.g., within a particular age group).
3. *Misclassification affected by the studied exposure.*

The methods of examination and classification regarding disease vary and influence accuracy (e.g., Feinstein 1985c). The extent of the misclassification is determined by the *sensitivity* of the method (the probability that a sick individual will be classified as sick) and the *specificity* (the probability that a healthy individual will be classified as healthy, in reference to the studied disease). The examination in terms of different variables (symptoms, signs, tests) may be more or less accurate. Diagnostic criteria and disease classification schemes vary by different degrees for different diseases. This may result in a nondifferential misclassification that is more or less pronounced depending on the disease. A similar effect arises if the disease has been given an overly broad definition—for example, pneumonia, if the exposure in question influences the risk of only certain types of pneumonia.

The relative risk is not influenced by an underdiagnosis (sensitivity <1) that is the same for the exposed and unexposed. If the comparison is based on incidence rate, one may obtain a certain diluting effect ($RR \rightarrow 1$), but this effect is negligible unless the incidence of the disease is high. In the case of an overdiagnosis (specificity <1) that is the same for the exposed and unexposed, the relative risk is influenced in the direction of $RR=1$ (e.g., White 1986). See Table 3.2.

TABLE 3.2. Misclassification with regard to disease
(nondifferential misclassification)

	Exposed	Unexposed	Relative risk
Number of individuals	2,000	8,000	
Number of cases	20	40	2.0
Underdiagnosis (sens. = 0.5, spec. = 1.0): Number identified as cases	10	20	2.0
Overdiagnosis (sens. = 1.0, spec. = 0.99): Number identified as cases	40	120	1.3

Misclassification influenced by a factor that is in covariance with the exposure may give an over- or underestimation of the relative risk. However, if such a factor is treated as a confounder in the investigation (for example, by stratification in the data analysis), the effect of such misclassification will always be an underestimation of the strength of the association (i.e., the relative risk is influenced in the direction of $RR = 1$). On the other hand, the relative risk after stratification is not always closer to the "true" value. (See, for example, Greenland, Robins 1985). In certain situations this type of misclassification may be reduced through restrictions in the choice of the study base.

Example 3.5: In an investigation of the association between exposure to soot and mortality from myocardial infarction, discussed in Example 3.2 and Example 3.4, chimney sweeps and other gainfully employed men aged 20 to 64 in 1960 were followed up with regard to death from myocardial infarction for a 20-year period. The men were consequently between the ages of 20 and 84 during the follow-up period. The accuracy of the information about specific cause of death is lower in the upper range of this age interval. In view of this, it may be suitable to make a separate comparison for the part of the study base for which the risk of misclassification is less, for example, the 20–64 age group.

The errors that arise if the misclassification is influenced by the studied exposure are the most serious. Such errors may lead to an over- or underestimation of relative risk that is impossible to correct in the data analysis. To avoid such misclassification, it may be necessary in certain situations for the diagnosis to be carried out blind (without knowledge of the exposure conditions) and for special measures to be taken to identify all cases that occur in the study base, whether they occasion contact with medical services or not. See Chapter 2.

OTHER SYSTEMATIC ERRORS

The choice of study base may, as mentioned previously, affect the validity of the investigation in terms of confounding and misclassification. The selection of a study population and follow-up period does not give rise to any other systematic errors, provided that the study population is defined prior to follow-up (Kleinbaum et al. 1981). *Nonparticipation,* however, deserves special attention. When subjects are lost to follow-up, this may introduce a systematic error in the investigation and result in an over- or underestimation of the relative risk (e.g., Criqui 1979). A similar error may arise if an open study population is defined in such a way that the exit of individuals from the study is related to the studied exposure and the occurrence of the disease. In certain case-control studies the choice of controls may introduce a systematic error (Chapter 9).

The study population should be defined at the start of the follow-up period. If the study population is defined only after the cases have occurred, the disease may affect the selection of the study population (*selection bias*). Assume, for example, that all individuals who visited a certain area 20 years ago were exposed. One now wants to investigate the occurrence of certain diseases among the exposed during the past 20 years. If there is an attempt, via the mass media or in another manner, to identify exposed individuals after the follow-up period, the selection may be influenced by the studied disease. (Those who fell ill may be more interested in participating in the investigation.) This can be avoided if the exposed individuals can instead be identified with the aid of a list of those who visited the area, drawn up 20 years ago (i.e., prior to follow-up).

SUBDIVISION OF SYSTEMATIC ERRORS

Systematic errors have often been subdivided into confounding, selection bias, and information bias (e.g., Kleinbaum et al. 1982). When this subdivision is applied, "information bias" is regarded as "selection bias" (and vice versa) if the study base is represented by a sample (case-control studies, Chapter 6). Furthermore, the defining of boundaries creates certain problems. Some common examples of selection bias in cohort studies have, for instance, fulfilled the criteria for confounding. The term *selection bias* has been occasionally used for systematic errors that are influenced by the selection of individuals (which in varying degrees applies to both confounding and misclassification), and the term *confounding* has sometimes been reserved for confounding that is (or could have been) controlled in the data analysis.

The subdivision of systematic errors that has been used here is based on the conditions in the study base, where the individuals may be misclassified regarding exposure or disease, and the comparability is influenced by confounding. In controlling confounding, any misclassification with respect to confounders should also be taken into account (e.g., Kupper 1984). This subdivision applies whether the whole study base is included (cohort studies) or whether it is represented by a random sample (Chapters 7 and 8). In case-control studies where the controls are selected in some other way (Chapter 9), they may not adequately represent the study base (misrepresentation), and this may result in an over- or underestimation of the relative risk.

4

Random Error

Random errors are those errors that involve a deviation from the true value in the individual investigation but would not lead to any average deviation from the true value if the investigation were repeated an infinite number of times with the same methodology. (Compare the hit pattern from a marksman with shaky hands but with a good rifle who "on average" hits the target.) *Precision* (reproducibility) is the absence of random errors.

Random errors arise on account of the investigation being based on a limited number of observations. Precision is improved (the random errors decrease) if a larger investigation is made, but this as a rule also increases the costs. The *efficiency* (cost-efficiency) of the investigation is the relation between precision and cost. Efficiency may be improved through the choice of study base, method of examination (for exposure and disease, respectively), and study design.

PRECISION

Random variation means that results based on a small number of observations are less reliable than results based on a large number of observations. In epidemiologic investigations the exposed individuals, as well as those who have fallen ill, are often a small proportion of all the individuals. The number of exposed cases, then, represents the smallest number of observations and consequently provides an idea of the precision of the study. Investigation results are often presented in the form of relative risks with, for example, a 95% confidence interval (e.g, Walker 1986a). The confidence interval provides information about the precision of the investigation. It is so constructed that, owing to random variations, the probability is 95%, for example, that it will cover the "true" value. The greater the number of observations, the tighter the confidence interval (greater precision).

When one is considering a confidence interval, its boundaries should not be regarded as rigid. The choice of a 95% interval is, in fact, disregarding tradition, an arbitrary choice. The assessment of the precision of the investigation is facilitated if one instead thinks of the point estimate (RR) surrounded by a series of confidence intervals, such as 99%, 95%, 90%, and 80%, where 99% is the widest and 80% is the tightest interval.

Precision can be improved by increasing the size of the study base, i.e., the number of subjects and/or the length of the follow-up period. [In case-control studies it is also possible, to a certain extent, to improve precision by increasing the number of controls (Chapter 6).] The desirability of a large-scale study that provides a high degree of precision must be weighed against the increased costs. First and foremost, various possibilities of improving precision without increasing the costs—i.e, improving the efficiency of the investigation—should be considered.

Once the optimal choices with regard to the efficiency and validity of the investigation have been made regarding the study design, source population, and method for the examination of the exposure conditions and follow-up of the disease occurrence, a decision should be reached on the size of the investigation. The question is often whether an available study base of a certain size would give "satisfactory" precision, provided that a certain association or no association between exposure and disease is found. If it is possible to estimate the exposure frequency and the incidence of the disease in the study base, it is possible to estimate a 95% confidence interval on the basis of various assumptions regarding the strength of the association, e.g., RR=1, RR=2, and RR=4 (or RR=0.5).

What should be considered a satisfactory precision is naturally a matter of judgment. However, if the relative risk shows a marked (or expected) association and the confidence interval contains RR=1, there is reason to question whether the precision of the investigation is sufficient. The same applies if RR=1 and the confidence interval contains marked associations. The alternatives then are to conduct a bigger study, to use a more efficient approach (in terms of study base, examination methods, or study design), or to refrain from carrying out the investigation.

In deciding on how big a study should be, a certain amount of guidance may be obtained from so-called power calculations. Moreover, certain foundations require that such calculations accompany applications for research grants. The "*power*" of an investigation is the probability of showing (as "statistically significant") an association of a certain strength (for example, RR=2 or RR=4) at a certain exposure frequency, significance level (for example, $p=0.05$), and study size (Casagrande et al. 1978). See Tables section.

Results of power calculations should be interpreted, however, with great caution. There are several reasons for this:

1. The result is an approximate estimation that depends on the significance level chosen (apart from tradition, this is an arbitrary choice) and on the estimates made with regard to the occurrence of the exposure and the strength of the association (which in practice are often unknown).
2. The result is an overestimation of the power of the investigation, since as a rule it does not account for nonparticipation (the extent of which may be difficult to forecast) and nondifferential misclassification (which occurs in nearly all investigations but is often impossible to forecast quantitatively).
3. The power (for example, 0.90 or 0.80) and, consequently, the study size that are suitable or acceptable is a matter of judgment.

(These limitations apply equally to the methods that have been described for estimating sample size requirement or smallest detectable RR for a certain study size.)

EFFICIENCY

A major problem with epidemiologic studies is that their precision is often low although they require major resources. Efficiency, i.e., the relation between precision and cost, may be improved, however, in several ways.

Precision is, as mentioned previously, often related to the number of cases of the disease that occur among the exposed. A small number of exposed cases (or a small number of unexposed cases) may result in too low a precision (wide confidence intervals) to provide sufficient information about the studied association. In many situations several tens of exposed cases are required for the investigation to give the desired precision. Table 4.1 shows the size of study base required for every ten exposed cases for a number of different diseases and exposure frequencies. The lower the incidence or exposure frequency, the bigger the required study base. Even for one of the most common types of cancer (colon cancer), the requirement is, for every ten exposed cases, more than 200,000 person-years at risk at 10% exposure frequency, or more than one million person-years at risk at 2% exposure frequency.

For a study to provide an adequate precision, it is necessary (except for the combination of high exposure frequency and high disease incidence) to follow a very large number of individuals over a long period. The resources required for this depend on: (1) the number of individuals; (2) the cost per individual for the examination and classification with respect to exposure conditions, including potential confounders; (3) the cost per year and individual for a follow-up regarding disease occurrence; (4) the length of the follow-up period; and (5) the cost of data handling and data analysis. Cohort studies are often major projects, both in terms of economic and

TABLE 4.1. *Size of study base required for every ten exposed cases (at RR=1) for certain diseases where the proportion of exposed in the study base is 50%, 10%, or 2%*

Disease (incidence rate)	Percentage of exposed in study base	Study base (number of person-years at risk) for every ten exposed cases
Myocardial infarction	50	2,300
$(8.7 \times 10^{-3}/\text{year})$	10	11,500
	2	57,500
Colon cancer	50	41,000
$(49.1 \times 10^{-5}/\text{year})$	10	204,000
	2	1,018,000
Lip cancer	50	221,000
$(9.0 \times 10^{-5}/\text{year})$	10	1,106,000
	2	5,529,000

Note: The study base is presumed to have an equal distribution among men aged 40–74 years. The incidence rates correspond to current Swedish rates.

personal contributions and from a purely administrative point of view. If, for example, the cost of the examination of exposure conditions is $100 per individual, the examination of 100,000 individuals costs $10 million. In addition to this are other costs, including the cost of, for example, 5 years of follow-up with respect to disease occurrence, which would give a maximum of 20 to 25 exposed cases of colon cancer (depending on mortality from other diseases) at RR=1 if the exposure frequency is 10% among men aged 40 to 74 years. Cohort studies of diseases with very high incidence require considerably fewer resources, particularly if the exposure frequency is high (close to 50% at RR=1).

There are various ways of improving the efficiency of the investigation depending on the association (exposure and disease) being studied.

Choice of Study Base

The efficiency of the study is influenced, as mentioned previously, by the exposure frequency and by the incidence of the disease and the strength of the association in the study base. These conditions may be influenced by the choice of study base.

Efficiency increases if a study base with a high exposure frequency (up to 50% at RR=1) is chosen. The occurrence of the studied exposure may vary among different age groups and geographical areas, for example, and the study base may be chosen with this in mind. If the exposure frequency is low, it is sometimes possible to increase efficiency considerably by choosing individuals from special groups of the population (for example, certain occupational groups) with a high exposure frequency. In certain situations some form of screening may be used to identify exposed individuals for more detailed examination and a follow-up of the disease occurrence. On the basis of the premises of a study, the optimal relationship between the number of exposed and unexposed individuals may be estimated (e.g., Morgenstern, Winn 1983). It may be advantageous to limit the investigation to highly exposed and unexposed individuals, if a stronger association at a higher exposure level is expected and if there is no wish to study the effect at different exposure levels.

The disease incidence may be higher in certain geographical areas or in certain age groups. The incidence rate given in Table 4.1 applies to men aged between 40 and 74 years. The incidence is higher in the upper part of the age interval. If the investigation is limited to men aged 60 to 74 years, the incidence rate for colon cancer, for example, increases to 88.8×10^{-5} per year and, as a result, the size of the study base required for a certain number of exposed cases decreases by almost half. The strength of the association (the relative risk) may vary, however, among different sections of the population—for example, different ages—and this may mean that a group with a high incidence is less suitable for a study of the effect of a certain exposure. If, for example, the difference in disease incidence between the exposed and unexposed is similar among younger and older men, the effect will be more obvious in the group that has the lower incidence, i.e., younger men. Overly tight restrictions in the choice of study base may lead to problems in identifying a sufficient number of individuals.

Examination of Exposure Conditions

The examination of exposure conditions can place very exacting demands on resources in cohort studies. Every reduction of the cost per individual means considerable savings if a large number of individuals are to be examined. Regarding choice of the examination method, the requirements are a low cost (to increase efficiency) and a high quality (to reduce misclassification with respect to exposure). These demands may result in a compromise between cost and quality. In the event of such a compromise, various examination methods should be compared in terms of: (1) the total cost (cost per individual $\times$ number of individuals) and (2) how the exposure misclassification can be expected to influence the result of the investigation (Chapter 3). Sometimes the choice of examination method can also influence the comparability and completeness of exposure information (Chapter 2). However, a simpler method of examination can introduce an error of the nondifferential misclassification type. In situations where a small or moderate error in the direction of $RR=1$ may be accepted, it may be possible to increase efficiency considerably by using a simpler and cheaper examination method (e.g., Byers et al. 1985).

Sometimes efficiency can be increased by comparing an exposed group with a sample of the population that is not being examined for exposure. This presupposes that the exposure frequency of the population is low (or at least known) and results in a certain underestimation of the strength of the association due to nondifferential misclassification (intermixture of exposed and unexposed individuals). A bigger problem may be the lack of information from the population sample about certain potential confounders (e.g., tobacco, alcohol).

Information about certain exposures is occasionally collected as a matter of routine or for other purposes and stored in an easily accessible form, such as computer-based registers. For such information to be usable in epidemiologic studies, it must be possible to identify the individuals (e.g., by means of a national registration number) in a manner that facilitates follow-up regarding disease occurrence. The use of a register may increase efficiency (decrease the cost) considerably, but it can also lead to certain validity problems in addition to those brought about by errors in the register: Information about certain potential confounders is often lacking, and information about the exposure in question may be of a low quality. The latter problem results, as a rule, in a nondifferential misclassification that leads to an underestimation of the strength of the association. The misclassification may be so great that it completely conceals an association. Certain registers (including, in Sweden, the National Census, the Cancer-Environment Registry, and the Cause-of-Death Registry) contain no information about specific occupational exposure; however, by combining information (on an individual basis) about occupation, branch of industry, professional status, etc., it is sometimes possible to identify groups with a very high or low exposure frequency. Such inclusion of the unexposed among the exposed and vice versa means that negative findings (i.e., when the relative risk appears to be close to unity) must be interpreted with great caution, but it does not constitute an objection to positive findings. Regardless of the findings, however, the lack of information about certain confounders may be a problem.

Follow-up of Disease Occurrence

Follow-up of disease occurrence in large studies often requires considerable resources, both administrative and financial. For certain diseases, however, there is a continuous, routine registration. In Sweden there are, for example, national registers of malignant tumor diseases (the Cancer Registry), congenital malformations (the Registry of Congenital Malformations), and mortality from specific diseases (the Cause-of-Death Registry). For several diseases registration exists regionally and locally. For certain diseases hospitalization registers may provide useful information. Naturally, it is necessary to distinguish morbidity (incidence) from, for example, medical care consumption. The proportion of cases that are diagnosed or that lead to hospitalization as a matter of routine vary almost between 0% and 100% for different diseases. Moreover, one case may give rise to several instances of medical care. Registers differ considerably in terms of quality and completeness. For certain diseases and causes of death, however, the registers may provide useful information and thus reduce considerably the cost of a follow-up of the disease occurrence.

Case-Control Design

In many situations a case-control design is the best way of improving the efficiency of the investigation. This applies particularly to diseases with a low incidence (Chapter 6).

5

Exercises for Chapters 1–4

1. The association between low to moderate alcohol consumption and the risk of developing a myocardial infarction among men of certain ages was investigated. Of 1,626 exposed and 1,840 unexposed men, 97 and 71, respectively, fell ill during the follow-up period. Smoking was considered a potential confounder in the study. A subdivision was therefore made into smokers and nonsmokers:

	Nonsmokers		Smokers	
	Exposed	Unexposed	Exposed	Unexposed
Disease	19	46	78	25
No disease	609	1,478	920	291
Total	628	1,524	998	316

Calculate the relative risk for exposed men (low to moderate alcohol consumption) versus unexposed men (no alcohol consumption):

a. Without considering smoking as a confounder.

b. Among nonsmokers.

c. Among smokers.

d. Did the investigation show any association between

low to moderate alcohol consumption and myocardial
infarction?

e. What measure of disease occurrence was used?

f. If smoking led to increased mortality, how would this
   influence the comparisons of parts *a, b,* and *c?*

g. If low to moderate alcohol consumption led to
   increased mortality, how would this influence the
   comparisons of parts *a, b,* and *c?*

2. In investigations aimed at describing the occurrence of a
   certain exposure, accuracy depends on the extent of
   misclassification, i.e., the method's sensitivity and specificity. In investigations aimed at comparing disease incidence among exposed and unexposed, accuracy is influenced to a high degree by the type of misclassification
   (Chapter 3). In a study population 10% are exposed, and
   90% are unexposed (true values). There is a simple and
   cheap examination method with sensitivity 0.5 and specificity 1.0. What effect does the misclassification have on
   the result of:

   a. An investigation aimed at describing the occurrence of
      exposure in the study population?

   b. An investigation aimed at studying the association
      between exposure and disease, if the misclassification
      is nondifferential and RR=2 (true relative risk)?

3. In a study, 2% of the exposed and 15% of the unexposed
   did not participate in the follow-up. If they had all participated in the follow-up, the study would have shown no
   association between exposure and the disease (RR=1).
   What result (RR) did the study show for those who were
   followed up, if the risk of developing the disease was twice

as high in those who did not participate compared with all the exposed and unexposed, respectively?

4. A cohort study is planned to investigate the association between an exposure whose occurrence is 25% and a disease whose incidence is 2.10^{-3} per year in the study base. How many person-years at risk should the study base include in order to give 30 exposed cases at RR=1? (Disregard any nonparticipation.)

5. What is the lowest exposure frequency at which one can expect to demonstrate (with power >0.9) an association between exposure and disease if RR=2 and a total of 200 cases (exposed plus unexposed) occur in a cohort study with a large study base? (See Tables section.)

6. In a cohort study, an investigation was made of the association between exposure to a drug (Bendectin, used for nausea) during pregnancy and pyloric stenosis (constriction of the opening from the stomach into the small intestine, with among other things, spurting vomiting) in children about 2–8 weeks after birth. This illness is more common among boys and possibly among first-born infants. About 300,000 members of a group health cooperative in Seattle obtained free medicines, which were registered together with information about childbirth and instances of medical care with diagnosis. During the period July 1, 1977, to June 30, 1982, 13,346 deliveries were registered among women who had been members for at least 280 days. Of these women, 3,835 had filled one or more prescriptions for Bendectin during pregnancy. Children of these women were classified as exposed, the remainder as unexposed. In the register 36 children were identified with pyloric stenosis, 29 of whom were born to mothers who had been members for at least 280 days. After examination of their medical records, three cases who did not fulfil the diagnostic criteria were excluded.

Pyloric stenosis was found in 13 of 3,835 exposed and in 13 of 9,511 unexposed infants, i.e. RR=2.5 (95% confidence interval 1.2–5.2).

a. Define the study base.

b. Why were women excluded who at the time of delivery had been members for less than 280 days?

c. What is the theoretically defined and empirically measured exposure? How may misclassification with respect to exposure have influenced the result?

d. Should one make a subdivision into several exposure categories? Which? What are the possibilities and limitations?

e. What measures should be taken to avoid misclassification with respect to disease?

f. Nausea (or factors associated with nausea) during pregnancy is an important potential confounder in the investigation. How would it be possible to avoid or control such confounding?

g. What other potential confounders should be taken into account?

7. An investigation was conducted to study the association between exposure to wood dust and development of various malignant tumors in the respiratory tract. In the Swedish National Census of 1960 there were, among men aged 20 to 64, a total of 8,141 furniture workers along with 1.4 million other gainfully employed workers. Those who developed cancer during the period 1961–79 were identified in the Cancer-Environment Register, which was established through a linkage between the National Census of 1960 and the Cancer Register. In the exposed

group, identification was made of, for example, 57 cases of lung cancer and 11 cases of adenocarcinoma in the nasal cavity. In the data analysis, stratification was made by year of birth and place of residence (county). The results showed no increased risk of lung cancer (RR=0.9, 90% confidence interval 0.7–1.1) or cancer of the larynx (RR=0.6, 0.3–1.4), but they revealed a substantial excess risk of adenocarcinoma in the nasal cavity and sinuses (RR=44.1, 26.6–68.9), particularly adenocarcinoma in the nasal cavity (RR=63.4, 35.5–104.9).

a. Define the study base.

b. What was the theoretically defined and empirically measured exposure?

c. What advantages and disadvantages will result from the means of classification with respect to exposure?

d. If the induction time was long, e.g., 10 years, how would this influence the result of the investigation?

e. What potential confounders have been taken into account in the investigation? In what way?

f. What other potential confounders should be taken into account?

g. How may the results have been influenced by any misclassification with respect to disease?

8. Against the background of low mortality from cardiovascular diseases among Eskimos in Greenland, a possible association between high fish consumption and low mortality rate from coronary heart disease was discussed. In 1960 a medical examination and dietary survey of a sample of 872 men between the ages of 40 and 59 years was conducted in Zutphen, a small town in the Nether-

lands. Information about dietary habits during the previous year was collected with a so-called dietary history method (which showed good agreement with chemical analyses of the diet in a sample of 49 men). Information was obtained about exposure (fish consumption) and potential confounders for 852 men who were then free of coronary heart disease. Of these, 78 men died from coronary heart disease during the 20-year follow-up period (no one was lost to follow-up):

Fish consumption (g/day)	Relative risk	95% confidence interval
0	1.00	
1–14	0.60	0.33–1.10
15–29	0.57	0.30–1.09
30–44	0.46	0.20–1.06
45+	0.42	0.16–1.13

a. Define the study base.

b. In many populations the vast majority have a moderate fish consumption and the proportion of those who do not eat fish is small. Among middle-aged men in Zutphen there was a relatively large proportion (20%) who did not eat fish and a similarly large proportion with a relatively high fish consumption. How does this affect the efficiency of this investigation?

c. Assume that the comparison was based on cumulative incidence and that mortality from other diseases increases with increasing fish consumption. How would this affect the result of the comparison? How can this be avoided?

d. The sample in 1960 included 872 men, but 20 of these were not involved in the follow-up. Why?

e. What potential confounders should be taken into account in the investigation?

f. Discuss the effect of any misclassification with respect to exposure or disease.

g. Discuss the precision of the results presented.

9. An association between human papilloma virus infection and development of cervical cancer (cancer of the neck of the womb) has been suggested. A gynecological health checkup in 1979 in Victoria, Australia, revealed 1,162 women whose smears showed abnormal epithelial cells suggestive of a human papilloma virus infection. Women were excluded whose smears showed evidence of concomitant herpes virus infection or dysplasia (which may develop into cervical cancer) or who showed previous evidence of dysplasia, carcinoma *in situ,* or invasive cervical cancer. All the women were recommended to have a repeat smear in 12 months, but 261 women did not turn up for a new checkup despite reminders. The remaining 846 women were followed up for cervical cancer (carcinoma *in situ*) using cervical smears (on average, 3.1 smears per woman) for up to 6 years, which gave 3,448 person-years at risk. A total of 30 cases of carcinoma *in situ* were identified among these exposed women. Age-specific incidence rates from the adjacent state of South Australia were used as estimates of the incidence of carcinoma *in situ* among unexposed women (notification to the Victorian Cancer Registry had been compulsory only since 1982). The relative risk was 15.6 (95% confidence interval 10.5–22.3).

a. Why were certain women excluded at the start of the follow-up period (1979)?

b. How are the 261 women who did not turn up for repeat examinations after 1979 to be regarded?

c. What was the follow-up period?

d. How many person-years were lost to follow-up among the exposed? How could this have influenced the result?

e. Discuss the choice of comparison group ("unexposed").

f. Could misclassification with respect to disease have influenced the result? In what way?

g. Could misclassification with respect to exposure have influenced the result? In what way?

10. Can physical activity prolong life? This question was the starting point for a cohort study of 16,936 men who, during the years 1916–50, entered Harvard College and who, in 1962 or 1966 (at ages of 35 to 74), answered a questionnaire on, among other things, physical activity. Questions such as how many city blocks they walked, how many stairs they climbed, and what types of sports they participated in and how much time they spent on them each week were used to assess the amount of physical activity (kcal/week). Information was also collected about other factors expected to influence mortality. The follow-up of mortality until 1978 (with less than 1% lost to follow-up) was limited to the ages 35 to 80 and covered 213,716 person-years and 1,413 deaths. After adjustment in the analysis for other factors found to influence mortality (age, smoking, hypertension, weight gain, parent's death before the age of 65), the relative risk was found to be 1.31 (95% confidence interval 1.15–1.49) for men with a low degree of physical activity (<2,000 kcal/week) compared with more active men. The relative risk for different levels of physical activity compared with the least active (<500 kcal/week) was 0.78 for 500–999 kcal/week, 0.73 for 1,000–1,499 kcal/week, 0.63 for 1,500–

1,999 kcal/week, 0.62 for 2,000–2,499 kcal/week, 0.52 for 2,500–2,999 kcal/week, 0.46 for 3,000–3,499 kcal/week, and 0.62 for ≥3,500 kcal/week. At ≥2,000 kcal/week life expectancy increased by 2.15 years on average compared with the lowest activity level (<500 kcal/week).

a. A potentially serious problem in the investigation is possible confounding from diseases (e.g., coronary heart disease) that may have influenced physical activity (1962/1966) and at the same time influenced mortality (during the period 1962–78 or 1966–78, respectively). How could one deal with this problem?

b. The association between physical activity and total mortality was investigated. High physical activity might, however, have different effects on mortality from different diseases. How could this influence the result of the investigation?

c. Misclassification with respect to exposure (physical activity) might arise, for example, if sufficient account was not taken of possible induction time. How would this influence the result of the investigation?

d. If physical activity does not prolong life, what is the most probable explanation of the observed association (apart from random variation)?

6

Principles of Case-Control Design

A *case-control study* (or case-referent study) is an investigation of the association between exposure and onset of disease, where use is made of exposure information from a sample of the study base ("controls"). The aim is to improve efficiency compared with the corresponding cohort study.

For the large majority of diseases, new cases occur at a relatively low rate. This means that the study base is, as a rule, very large in relation to the number of cases (see, for example, Table 4.1). The cohort design is therefore often inefficient. The principle of a case-control study is that information on exposure (and potential confounders) from a representative sample of the study base replaces information from the whole study base. As a result, efficiency can be considerably improved, particularly in studies of diseases with a low or moderate incidence.

Figure 6.1 shows the principle behind a case-control study in relation to the corresponding cohort study. As in the cohort study, a study base and all cases of the disease that occur in the study base are identified. A sample ("controls") is then drawn with the purpose of obtaining information on the exposure frequency in the study base. For the data analysis, only information from cases and controls is used. The relative risk, i.e., the ratio of the incidence of the disease among the exposed and the unexposed, is estimated by:

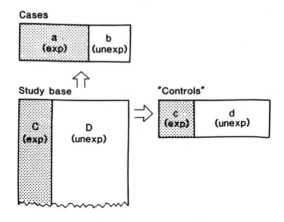

Cohort study:

Relative risk (RR) = $\dfrac{\text{incidence among exposed}}{\text{incidence among unexposed}} = \dfrac{a/C}{b/D} \left(= \dfrac{aD}{bC}\right)$

Case–control study:

Relative risk (RR) = $\dfrac{ad}{bc}$

FIG. 6.1. Principles of cohort design and case-control design.

$$RR = \frac{ad}{bc}$$

with the following designations:

	Exposed	Unexposed
Cases	a	b
Controls	c	d

When the study population is open, the comparison is based on *incidence rate*. The controls will then be selected so that they represent the total person-time in the study base. This means that controls are selected continuously during the follow-up period or as the cases occur. In this way, account is taken of changes in the composition of the study base, with respect to exposure and potential confounders, due to individuals moving into and out of the study population during the follow-up period. The controls represent person-years (not individuals) in the study base, which means, for example, that individuals who fall ill can be selected as controls before they fall ill (Lubin, Gail 1984)—and after they have recovered, if the investigation covers recurring onsets of the disease.

Even when the study population is a closed one, the comparison is usually based on incidence rate. The controls are then selected in the same way as when the study population is open. Account is thus taken of changes in the composition of the study base owing to mortality (and occurrence of the studied disease) during the follow-up period. Again, the controls represent person-years (not individuals) in the study base.

When the study population is a closed one, the comparison is sometimes based on *cumulative incidence.* The study base is then replaced by the study population: Controls are selected among the individuals included in the study at the start of the follow-up period and thus represent individuals (not person-years). In a comparison of this kind, account is not taken, however, of any differences in mortality (or occurrence of the studied disease) between the exposed and unexposed (cf. the procedure for cohort studies, Chapter 2). In case-control studies where the comparison is based on cumulative incidence, controls are often selected among the subjects in the study population who have not fallen ill during the follow-up period ("non-cases"). This affords certain advantages in the data analysis. Provided that only a small proportion of the study population fall ill ("rare disease assumption"), controls selected in this manner provide an estimate of the exposure frequency in the study population (e.g., Schlesselman 1982). There is much to suggest, however, that controls should be selected from the whole study population (Miettinen 1985a).

Case-control studies, like cohort studies, are consequently aimed at comparing the disease incidence among exposed and unexposed. Using the principle in Fig. 6.1 as the starting point, case-control studies may be designed in different ways. In two of the designs that will be described here (Chapters 7 and 8), controls are selected as a random sample of the study base (or study population); in the third (Chapter 9), controls are selected in another manner. In one design (Chapter 7), primary exposure information is collected before the cases occur; in the remaining two designs (Chapters 8 and 9), information is collected only after the cases have occurred. (Regarding the subdivision of epidemiologic investigations, see Chapter 11.) The choice of study design has different consequences for validity and efficiency in different situations.

Whether the controls are selected as a random sample of the study base or in another manner, the question sometimes arises of whether the controls should be matched to the cases. One possibility is *individual matching,* i.e., for each case a selection is made of one control (matched pairs), two controls, etc. that are similar to the case in terms of one or possibly more potential confounders (e.g., age). Another possibility is to subdivide the study base into a number of strata with respect to one or more potential confounders (e.g., different age groups), after which the size of the sample from each stratum is chosen in relation to the proportion of cases in the respective stratum, e.g., a similar number of controls as cases in every age group (*frequency matching*). A matching of controls to cases does not mean that exposed and unexposed individuals become alike with respect to the factor (confounder, e.g., age) concerned in the matching and therefore does not lead to control of confounding (see, for example, Axelson 1985a). The aim is instead to improve the efficiency of the investigation. Increased efficiency is achieved if there is a strong association between the matching factor and the studied disease, particularly if the matching factor has a low frequency in the study base. Otherwise there is usually little or no improvement of efficiency. If the factor in question is in covariance with the exposure but is not a risk indicator for the disease in the study base, matching leads instead to a decrease in efficiency (*overmatching*). Matching may also lead to certain other problems. An example is nonparticipation in studies with matched pairs where the pairs are kept together in the data analysis, which leads to the whole pair dropping out if information from a case or control is lacking. Matching based on a certain factor (e.g., age) means, in addition, that the investigation cannot be utilized for studying how this factor influences the risk of falling ill. Consequently, even if matching may be motivated to improve the efficiency of the investigation, there are several reasons for showing restraint with matching in case-control studies (e.g., Howe, Choi 1983).

How many controls should be selected? This depends on (1) the number of cases and (2) the resources required for increasing the number of controls or the size of the study base (and, consequently, the number of cases). A study with a certain number of cases produces a higher precision the more controls that are selected. This effect is, however, increasingly marginal with an increasing number of controls. If the number of controls is equal to the number of cases, the study yields approximately 50% of the theoretically maximum precision (with an infinite number of controls). If the number of controls is four times the number of cases, the study yields about 80% of the maximum precision. The proportion of the theoretically maximum precision is approximately $r/(r+1)$, where r=number of controls/number of cases. Figure 6.2 shows how the number of controls affects both precision and the cost of examining the controls in a case-control study with a fixed number of cases. In practice, there is seldom or never a motivation for selecting more than four or five times as many controls as cases. In many situations the most efficient solution is to select the same number of controls as cases. On the basis of the premises of a study, it is possible to estimate the relationship between the number of controls and the number of cases that is optimal from the point of view of efficiency (e.g., Morgenstern, Winn 1983).

Some conception of the efficiency of a case-control study in relation to the corresponding cohort study may be obtained by comparing Table 6.1 with Table 4.1. In many situations, several tens of exposed cases are required for the investigation to produce the desired precision. Regarding study size and power, see the Tables section at the back of the book.

In regard to the identification of different sources of systematic errors, the conditions discussed earlier for cohort studies (Chapter 3) also apply to case-control studies. In

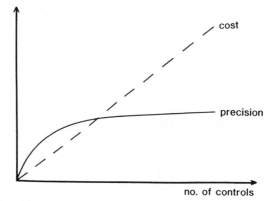

FIG. 6.2. Precision and cost of examining the controls in relation to the number of controls used in a case-control study with a fixed number of cases, where the cost of examining each control is independent of the number of controls examined.

certain case-control studies there are additional potential sources of systematic errors (Chapters 8 and 9).

The case-control design means that the lower the incidence of the studied disease and the higher the cost of obtaining information on exposure (including potential confounders), the higher the potential efficiency compared with the corresponding cohort study. Sometimes the efficiency can be increased by utilizing the same control group in two (or more) case-control studies (with the same study base) of different diseases that are of interest in relation to the studied exposure conditions.

TABLE 6.1 *Number of individuals (cases plus controls) required for every ten exposed cases (at RR = 1) in a case-control study*

Percentage of exposed in the study base	Number of individuals	
	$r=1$	$r=4$
50	40	100
10	200	500
2	1,000	2,500

$r=$ number of controls/number of cases.

7

Case-Control Design A

In the type A case-control study, controls are selected at random from the study base, and primary information on exposure is collected before the cases occur.

STUDY DESIGN

Type A case-control studies are similar to most cohort studies in that the primary information on exposure is collected prior to follow-up from all subjects in the study population (which, as a rule, is a closed population). However, this primary information is further analyzed only for the cases and a random sample of the study base.

When all the subjects in the study population have been examined with respect to exposure conditions, the information is stored in the form of unprocessed data. This means that questionnaires are completed, checked for completeness and supplemented where necessary, and then stored without the primary data being encoded, transferred to another form (e.g., magnetic tape), or processed in any way (e.g., classified in terms of exposure by combining information from different questions). Similarly, the results of measurements and observations are kept in the form of raw, unprocessed data. Specimens are stored with no preceding analysis, provided that the storage costs do not exceed the analysis costs, if this can be done in a way (e.g., freezing of blood specimens) that allows a selection of the specimens to be analyzed at the end of the follow-up period.

A follow-up with respect to the disease incidence is carried out in the same way as in cohort studies. For the disease(s) being studied, all cases that occur in the study base should be identified.

Controls are selected at random from the study base (as an independent random sample or by frequency or individual matching of controls to the cases). For all the cases and controls, the questionnaires and measurement/observation results are identified for encoding and processing, and specimens are identified for analysis. All handling of primary data is carried out blind (i.e., without knowledge of case-control status), and the information is passed on in a suitable form for data analysis.

VALIDITY

A type A case-control study differs in principle in only one respect from the corresponding cohort study: Information from the whole study base is replaced by information from a random sample of the study base. A potential source of error is the way in which the sampling is carried out. To avoid such errors, the sampling frame must cover the whole study base (but only the study base), and strict rules must be applied in carrying out the sampling. This is, however, a technical problem; the principles for random sampling are described in textbooks on statistics.

If the investigation involves the storage of specimens (e.g., frozen blood specimens), there is naturally a possibility of the specimens being ruined or of their quality deteriorating during storage. In certain situations it may be of interest to use exposure information collected earlier for other purposes, for example, examination results from a health check or work environment investigation. If 100% of these primary data have not been saved, the possibility should be considered that the information lost is related to exposure and disease. This would introduce a systematic error that may lead to an over- or underestimation of the relative risk. Similar problems may, however, also arise in cohort studies.

All other conditions for validity of type A case-control studies are the same as for most cohort studies (Chapter 3). The difference from the corresponding cohort study does not apply to validity but to precision and cost (efficiency). This difference, however, may be regulated by means of the size of the sample of the study base (i.e., the number of controls). Should the sample represent 100% of the study base, the investigation would be equivalent to a cohort study (see, for instance, Example 7.1).

EFFICIENCY

Compared with the corresponding cohort study, the type A case-control study means a saving in resources corresponding to the cost of the analysis of specimens; encoding and processing of information from questionnaires, measurements, and observations; and making the information analyzable (e.g., by transferring it to magnetic tapes). The extent of the savings depends on the cost per individual and the difference between the number of subjects in the study population and the number of controls. Sometimes other costs, such as those arising from the storage of specimens, must also be taken into account. If a large number of controls is selected, the precision achieved approaches that of the corresponding cohort study. The number of controls should, however, be chosen with regard both to cost and to precision (see Chapter 6).

Example 7.1: A study was planned to investigate how certain blood lipids influence the risk of developing colon cancer. The cost of the analysis of a blood specimen was estimated at US $50 and the incidence of colon cancer at 49×10^{-5} per year (men 40 to 74 years of age). Blood specimens from a study population of 40,000 men were drawn and frozen with no preceding analyses. Those who developed colon cancer during the next 10 years were identified via a national cancer register.

From a list of the study population, controls were selected by means of individual age matching to the cases. Information about deaths during the follow-up period was collected to take into account differences in mortality. The frozen blood specimens (and information about certain potential confounders) were identified in all 200 cases and in a similar number of controls. The total cost of the analysis of the blood specimens was put at US $20,000 and achieved about 50% of the maximum precision (Chapter 6). If twice as many controls were chosen, the costs would increase to US $30,000 and the information yield to 67% of the maximum precision. The cost of a corresponding cohort study was estimated at US $40,000×50=US $2 million. Provided that the frozen specimens are not damaged (or saved selectively), the case-control design does not introduce any systematic errors compared with the corresponding cohort study.

Example 7.2: In an investigation of the association between workload and the occurrence of backache, 4,000 young men employed for certain installation work (and with no history of backache) were examined with regard to, among other things, working positions and loads. Extensive exposure information was stored in the form of raw data. During the follow-up period, 200 men developed backache. For every case, four controls were selected at random from the study base. At the end of the follow-up period, the exposure information from the cases and controls was encoded, processed, and transferred to a suitable form for data analysis. This was done blind, i.e., without knowledge of which were cases and which were controls. The cost of encoding and processing was put at US $10 per individual, i.e., a total of US $10,000 for 200 cases and 800 controls. This yielded about 80% of the maximum precision. The corresponding cost of a cohort study was put at US $4,000×10=US $40,000.

8

Case-Control Design B

In the type B case-control study, controls are selected at random from the study base, and exposure information is collected only after the cases have occurred.

STUDY DESIGN

Type B case-control studies are similar to type A case-control studies in that controls are selected as a random sample of the study base. However, exposure information is collected only from the cases and controls. Thus, exposure information is collected only after the cases have been identified. The study population is often, but not always, an open population.

The first stage is, as in the study designs described earlier (Chapters 2 and 7), definition of the study base. Whether the study population is an open or a closed one, the study base must be available for random sampling (via a sampling frame, for example, a current population register), and the individuals in the sample must be available for examination with respect to exposure conditions, including potential confounders. In addition, it should be possible to identify all cases of the studied disease that occur in the study base.

Selection of the study base, as well as preparation of the measuring instruments, questionnaires, and examination routines, is done before the start of the follow-up period. Unlike the study designs described previously however, exposure information is not collected before the start of the follow-up period. The next step is instead a follow-up with respect to disease onset: All the cases occurring in the study base are identified. Then they are examined regarding exposure conditions, including potential confounders. As the cases are identified, controls are selected at random from the study base (as an independent random sample, or by means of frequency or individual matching of controls to the cases) and examined regarding exposure conditions, including potential confounders. Information from the cases and controls is encoded, processed, and transferred to a suitable form for data analysis.

In some countries, such as the Scandinavian ones, the conditions are favorable for population-based case-control studies of this type because of, among other things, well-run population registers as well as registers of disease incidence (e.g., cancer registers) and defined catchment areas in the medical service sector.

VALIDITY

The study design described here differs from the one described in the previous chapter in terms of the time for obtaining the primary exposure information. This may influence validity since it opens up the possibility that the disease may influence the classification with regard to exposure (Chapter 3). Measurements (e.g., blood pressure) and observations from the cases will always be based on the conditions after the onset of the disease. If they have been changed because of the disease, a systematic error is introduced into the investigation. No such error, however, arises in connection with measurements and observations that are not influenced by the disease.

As for interview and questionnaire data, the situation in this respect is more favorable: The questions can be formulated so that they refer to conditions before the onset of the disease. If the disease influences answers, however, errors of this type can still arise. This may occur (1) if the people who fall ill suspect that there is an association (for example, based on information via the mass media) or (2) if the disease has led to changes in the exposure conditions, and this influences the reporting of previous exposure (e.g., Persson, Norell 1989). Moreover, it has been maintained that sick individuals (irrespective of the disease) generally differ from healthy people ("population controls") in their answers to questions about previous exposure. Empirical data do not suggest, however, that this is a serious problem (e.g., Norell, Ahlbom 1987).

Whether or not the disease may be expected to influence the exposure information naturally depends on the association (exposure and disease) that is being studied. It is sometimes necessary to take special measures to minimize the risk of this, for example, by interviewing the cases immediately after or even before a definite diagnosis. (An approach that is occasionally used is comparison with the "preliminary cases" that have been given another, final diagnosis.) It may be possible to ask at the end of the interview whether the subject knows of the studied association and whether the exposure conditions have changed.

For certain measurements (for example, blood pressure) and observation [for example, examination of X-ray pictures or microscopic preparations (see Example 8.2)], the results may be influenced by the examiner's knowledge of the aim of the study. To avoid this, the investigation of the exposure conditions should, whenever possible, be conducted blind, i.e., without knowledge of case-control status.

The systematic error that arises if the disease influences classification in terms of exposure may lead to an over- or underestimation of the relative risk that is impossible to correct in the data analysis. If this is a potential problem in the investigation, careful consideration should be given to suitable measures in the collection of data. Type A case-control studies avoid this problem, but their efficiency as a rule is considerably lower.

In studies of an association (exposure-disease) with a long induction time, exposure information that reflects the conditions immediately before the onset of the disease, may differ from the conditions during an earlier (etiologically relevant) period, and this may introduce a nondifferential misclassification. A corresponding problem in cohort studies is where the exposure information reflects the conditions at the start of the follow-up period.

Among those who have been separately identified as cases and controls, there will nearly always be subjects who cannot be examined with respect to exposure conditions. If such non-participation is related to the exposure, the examined cases will not reflect the exposure frequency among all the cases, and the examined controls will not reflect the exposure frequency in the study base. This introduces a systematic error that may lead to over- or underestimation of the relative risk (unless the nonparticipation removes similar proportions of the exposed and the unexposed from both cases and controls).

Other conditions that apply with regard to validity are the same as for the study designs previously described (Chapters 3 and 7).

To save time, it is sometimes possible to identify a study population in the past (e.g., from census data) and to identify the cases (e.g., from a cancer register) for a follow-up period in the past. Cases and controls will then be examined for exposure conditions only after the follow-up period. This may, however, increase the problems of differential misclassification discussed previously. In addition, some of the cases and controls may have died, and one may have to rely on exposure information obtained from relatives or other informants.

EFFICIENCY

The collection of data is limited to cases and controls. This means a savings in resources over previously described designs corresponding to the cost of data collection and handling for the rest of the study base. Regarding precision, the same conditions apply as for type A case-control studies. Efficiency may therefore be very high, particularly if the exposure frequency is moderate or high and the incidence of the disease is low.

Example 8.1: A case-control study was planned to investigate how estrogen (female sex hormone) and certain dietary factors influence the risk of fracture of the neck of the femur (hip fracture) in women aged 50 to 79. At five major hospitals with defined catchment areas, identification was made of all cases of this fracture diagnosed among women of these ages and resident in the catchment areas during a 2-year period. Standardized interviews were conducted concerning previous exposure (for example, estrogen treatment, oophorectomy, certain dietary factors) and potential confounders. Every month interviews were conducted in the same way with an identical number of controls among women of the ages in question, selected as an age-stratified random sample from current population registers for the different catchment areas.

Example 8.2: The occurrence of dysplastic nevi (pigment patches in the skin) is considered to increase the risk of malignant melanoma (a malignant skin tumor). A case-control study was planned to investigate this—and, consequently, the prospects of removing dysplastic nevi as a preventive measure. All individuals aged 20 to 79 who had been given the diagnosis of malignant melanoma during a four-year period were identified via a special melanoma unit, to which all cases of the disease that were diagnosed within a defined catchment area were referred for examination. Controls were selected every 6 months as an age-stratified random sample among individuals of the ages 20 to 79 taken from a current population register for the catchment area. Every month a similar number of cases and controls were examined with respect to the presence of dysplastic nevi (clinical and histopathological examination). Special measures were taken so that the examination could be conducted blind, i.e., without the examiner knowing which subjects were cases and which were controls.

9

Case-Control Design C

In the type C case-control study, controls are selected in a different way (not at random from the study base), and exposure information is collected only after the cases have occurred.

STUDY DESIGN

Type C case-control studies are similar to type B studies in that exposure information is collected only from the cases and controls—thus, only after the cases have been identified. However, unlike the case-control studies described previously (Chapters 7 and 8), the controls are not selected at random from the study base.

A common reason for this is that the cases were selected in such a way that the corresponding study base is not available for random sampling. This occurs, for example, if all the cases diagnosed at a hospital during the follow-up period are selected, but only a portion of the individuals in the catchment area falling ill during this period are diagnosed at the hospital (e.g., some are diagnosed and handled in the primary medical care service, and others do not visit a doctor at all). The study base can then be theoretically defined on the basis of the individuals who would have been diagnosed at the hospital if they had fallen ill during the follow-up period. Such a (conceptual) study base is, however, not available for random sampling.

In certain situations, even if the study base is available for random sampling, controls are selected in another way. One reason may be the attempt to improve comparability between cases and controls in terms of the quality of the exposure information. Another reason may be the expectation that the participation rate in the examination of exposure conditions (which may include time-consuming or unpleasant procedures) would be unacceptably low among controls selected at random from the study base but considerably higher among controls selected in another manner.

The controls may be selected from, for example, (1) other patients treated in the same hospital (hospital controls), (2) subjects who have died (dead controls), or (3) neighbors, siblings, and others related to the cases (neighbor controls). Regarding design and implementation, this type of case-control study in all other respects matches a type B case-control study.

VALIDITY

In contrast to type A and type B case-control studies, the choice of controls is one of the main problems for the type C case-control study. The task of the controls is to reflect the exposure frequency in the study base that generated the cases. If hospital controls are chosen, the following points should therefore be taken into account:

1. If the exposure influences the risk of developing the disease(s) afflicting the controls, a systematic error is introduced into the investigation. It is therefore unsuitable to choose, for example, patients with chronic bronchitis and certain other respiratory diseases as controls in a study of the association between smoking and myocardial infarction. Many exposures (tobacco, alcohol, fat consumption, etc.) may influence the risk of contracting any of a large number of diseases. If several exposures of this kind are studied, it may be difficult to choose suitable hospital controls.

2. If the exposure influences the probability of those who develop the disease(s) afflicting the controls being identified at the hospital, a systematic error is introduced into the investigation—unless this effect is identical for cases and controls. It may in practice be difficult to achieve similarity between cases and controls in this respect (the probability of hospital care varies almost between 0 and 100% for different diseases), particularly if the controls are selected among instances of hospitalization for several diseases.

The latter problem may require particular consideration. If, for example, subjects with arthrosis are more likely to be hospitalized if they also have a raised blood pressure, patients being treated for arthrosis are an unsuitable control group in a study of the association between hypertension and myocardial infarction (even if hypertension does not influence the risk of developing arthrosis).

In case-control studies where (some of) the cases are dead when they are examined with respect to exposure, the possibility of selecting dead controls for dead cases may be considered. The aim is to achieve comparability in terms of the quality of the exposure information and, consequently, a misclassification that is independent of the disease. The problem is that the individuals in the study base who die (from other causes) may not reflect the exposure frequency in the study base, which consists of the living (e.g., McLaughlin et al. 1985a,b). If the exposure influences the risk of dying from the cause(s) of death in the controls—or the probability of these being identified—a systematic error is introduced into the investigation (cf. hospital controls). If appreciable differences between living and dead individuals with respect to the quality of the exposure information are not expected, there is, as a rule, no reason for selecting dead controls. Sometimes, however, the possibility of examining exposure conditions is influenced by whether the individuals are alive or dead (see Example 9.2).

If neighbor controls are chosen, validity depends on the

extent to which they reflect the exposure frequency in the (conceptual) study base. When the cases are selected in such a way that the study base is not available for random sampling, such controls may be no better in that respect than a random sample of the population in the catchment area. The study can then be compared with a type B case-control study in which it is not possible to identify all the cases, but only those that were hospitalized, which may introduce a systematic error into the study.

A case-control study may embrace several exposures and potential confounders, and the possibility that systematic errors may be introduced through the choice of controls must be considered for every exposure being studied. When it is suspected that the choice of controls may introduce a systematic error, the choice of another study design may be considered. If the study base is available for random sampling but hospital controls are selected with the aim of improving comparability in terms of the quality of exposure information, two control groups may be selected: hospital controls and a random sample of the study base, which are kept separate in the data analysis. If the study base is not available for random sampling, consideration may be given to selecting the cases in another manner so that the study base is available.

The selection of cases determines the study base (or vice versa) and, consequently, the difficulties of finding a suitable control group. In other respects, the conditions for validity are the same as those that apply in a type B case-control study (Chapter 8).

EFFICIENCY

In regard to the efficiency of the investigation, in the main the same conditions apply as for a type B case-control study. In certain situations it is possible to achieve even greater efficiency, because it may be easier to identify the cases (and perhaps also to examine the controls). This presupposes, however, that a suitable control group can be found.

Example 9.1: An investigation was planned to study how certain psychological factors influence the risk of middle-aged women developing a myocardial infarction. The aim was to study all the women of age 40 to 64 who had received the diagnosis of myocardial infarction at two hospitals with defined catchment areas. The examination included extensive interviews and psychological tests as well as clinical and laboratory examinations with respect to potential confounders. For several reasons a relatively low participation rate was expected among controls selected at random from the study base. As a result, the question arose as to whether the controls examined would reflect the exposure frequency in the study base. Against this background, the possibility was discussed of selecting controls among patients with one or several other diagnoses in the two hospitals.

Example 9.2: Air pollutants in the form of fibers, which occur in certain working environments and housing, are assumed to increase the risk of malignant mesothelioma (a malignant tumor disease). A case-control study was planned to investigate how the fiber concentration in the lung tissues influences the risk of developing malignant mesothelioma. Specimens, consisting of lung tissue for examination in an electron microscope, were collected during operations or autopsies from all men in a geographically defined population who during a 10-year period had received a diagnosis of malignant mesothelioma. As the cases were identified, age-matched controls in the population in question were selected among men who died of other diseases and were subjected to autopsies. The examination of the lung tissue was conducted blind.

10

Exercises to Chapters 6–9

11. An investigation was planned concerning the association between certain dietary factors and hip fractures. The intent was to study the effect of current dietary habits as well as those 5 years previously, using standardized interviews. The following alternatives were discussed:

    I.   Type A case-control study—or a cohort study—in which information about current dietary habits is collected 5 years before and immediately preceding the start of the follow-up period.

    II. Type A case-control study—or a cohort study—in which information about current dietary habits as well as those 5 years previously is collected immediately before the start of the follow-up period.

    III. Type B case-control study in which information about current dietary habits and those 5 years previously is collected as the cases are identified.

    IV. Type C case-control study in which information about dietary habits is collected in the same way as in alternative III.

    a. In what respects does a cohort study (in alternative I or

II) differ from a corresponding type A case-control study in terms of validity and efficiency?

b. In what respects does alternative II differ from alternative I in terms of validity and efficiency? How does this influence the result of the investigation?

c. In what respects does alternative III differ from alternative II in terms of validity and efficiency? How does this influence the result of the investigation?

d. In what respects does alternative IV differ from alternative III in terms of validity and efficiency? How does this influence the result of the investigation?

e. Which study design should one choose, taking into account the validity and efficiency of the investigation?

12. Example 7.1 described a type A case-control study of how certain blood lipids influence the risk of developing colon cancer. What problems may be expected if the investigation were instead designed as a type B case-control study?

13. Example 8.2 described an investigation of the association between dysplastic nevi and malignant melanoma.

a. Define the study base.

b. Was the study population open or closed?

c. What potential confounders (apart from age and sex) should be taken into account?

d. Could the exposure influence classification with respect to the studied disease (malignant melanoma)? In what direction would this influence the relative risk?

e. Could the disease influence classification with respect to exposure (dysplastic nevi)? In what direction would this influence the relative risk?

f. The possibility of designing the investigation as a type A case-control study was discussed. What advantages and disadvantages would this have?

g. The possibility of designing the investigation as a type C case-control study was discussed. What advantages and disadvantages would this have?

14. Example 9.1 described an investigation of the association between certain psychological factors and the risk of developing a myocardial infarction. What requirements should be placed on hospital controls?

15. At the department of ophthalmology of a university hospital, a case-control study was planned to investigate the association between certain types of radiation and cataract development. The cases consisted of patients who during a 2-year period were diagnosed at the department as having a cataract and were resident in its catchment area. Cataracts are more common among older people, and the investigation was limited to individuals 65 to 79.

a. Define the study base.

b. How should the controls be selected?

c. Discuss different alternatives regarding the design of a case-control study.

16. Exercise 6 (Chapter 5) described a cohort study of exposure to a drug (Bendectin) during pregnancy and its association with pyloric stenosis in the infant during the first

months after birth. There was an interest in subdividing the exposure on the basis of different time periods during pregnancy and in controlling certain confounders that were not identifiable in the registers. This would require an extensive examination of the records of the 13,346 infants who were included in the study population. To improve the efficiency of the investigation, a sample was drawn from the study population. In this way, the examination of the records could be limited to the sample (controls) and the cases.

a. Is the study population open or closed?

b. Is it available for random sampling?

c. What should be taken into account regarding the question of the sample size, i.e., the number of controls?

d. What can be gained by matching controls to cases on the basis of, for example, sex?

e. What should be borne in mind with regard to the quality of the medical records about, for example, the length of gestation and smoking habits during pregnancy?

f. What type of case-control study is this?

17. The association between passive smoking and lung cancer was investigated in a case-control study of Swedish women. From two major surveys about smoking habits in two different population samples (1961 and 1963), a total of 27,409 women were identified who had never smoked. In the National Cancer Register and Cause-of-Death Register, 92 cases of lung cancer were identified among these women through 1980. On examination of the medical records, the diagnosis of primary lung cancer was verified for 77 cases, 24 of which had squamous or small-

cell carcinomas (which have the strongest association with smoking). For every case four age-matched controls were selected.

In a new survey (1984) supplemented with telephone interviews with cases and controls (or with next of kin, except husband, for the women who had died), the husbands' smoking habits were examined for the women who had been married. Information on potential confounders was also obtained. The participation rate was 90% among the cases and 96% among the controls. For women who had been married to smokers (compared with women who were unmarried or married to non-smokers) the relative risk was 3.3 (95% confidence interval 1.1–11.4) for squamous and small-cell carcinoma, and 0.8 (0.4–1.5) for other primary lung cancers. A subdivision was made into high exposed (the husband had smoked >15 cigarettes/day or 50 g pipe tobacco/ week during at least 30 years of marriage) and low exposed (other exposed individuals). The relative risk of squamous and small-cell carcinoma was 6.4 (1.1–34.7) for high exposed and 1.8 (0.6–5.3) for low exposed.

a. Define the study base. Is the study population open or closed? What type of case-control study is this?

b. Why was the investigation limited to women who had never smoked? How could the information from 1961/63 be supplemented in this respect?

c. What is the theoretically defined and empirically measured, respectively, exposure? Discuss potential sources of misclassification with respect to exposure.

d. Misclassification with respect to disease was a potential problem in the investigation. Assume that 14 of 20 examined cases with squamous or small-cell carcinoma and 40% of the corresponding controls were exposed (RR=3.5). How would the relative risk be

influenced if added to these cases were the 15 cases
that were identified in the registers but whose diagnosis had not been verified (if RR=1 for these)? How
would the relative risk be influenced if added to the 20
cases were 50 cases of verified primary lung cancer of
another type (if RR=1 for these)?

e. What potential confounders (apart from age) should
be taken into account in the investigation?

18. Does overweight increase the risk of breast cancer? A
case-control study in Israel was based on all newly diagnosed breast cancer patients (cases) and, for each case, a
patient with nonmalignant, nongastrointestinal, nongy-
necologic disease ("surgical control"), identified among
19 surgical wards of the eight major hospitals in the Tel
Aviv area, 1975–78. In addition, voting lists were used to
select a "neighborhood control" for each case, living in
the same or an adjacent voting area. Information on
recent weight (for cases and surgical controls before
illness began), height, and potential confounders was
obtained by interview. Response rates were 96% for cases
and surgical controls and 72% for neighborhood controls.
Subjects were divided into the following categories
according to body mass index [BMI=weight (kg)/height
(m)^2]: ≤19 ("unexposed"), 19.1–23, 23.1–27, and ≥27.1.
The relative risk at each level of exposure (among women
aged 60+) was respectively, 1.17, 1.44, and 2.38, using
information from the surgical controls, and 1.78, 1.92,
and 2.53, using information from the neighborhood
controls.

a. What type of case-control study is this? Is the selection
of controls a problem in this study?

b. Why were patients with malignant, gastrointestinal,
and gynecologic diseases not included among the
surgical controls?

c. What are the advantages of using surgical controls and neighborhood controls, respectively?

d. Discuss the importance of potential sources of misclassification with respect to exposure.

e. What potential confounders, except age, should one take into account in the investigation?

19. To investigate whether a low intake of vitamin A increases the risk of stomach cancer, a study was carried out based on deceased cases and controls. Registers were used for the identification of all individuals in a certain part of Pennsylvania who died of stomach cancer in 1978–79. Controls were selected among subjects who died from a cause related to arteriosclerotic heart disease in the same area during the same years, and these were matched to the cases (e.g., by age and sex). Information about dietary habits and other pertinent factors was collected blind through telephone interviews with the next of kin. The nonresponse rate was 27.5% among the cases (42 of 153 individuals) and 23 6% among the controls. For a vitamin A intake below 5,000 IU/day, the relative risk was 1.7 (95% confidence interval 1.0–3.1).

a. What type of case-control study is this?

b. Why were dead controls chosen? Can the choice of controls introduce a systematic error into the investigation?

c. The nonresponse rate in the interviews was fairly high. Assume that the exposure frequency among the examined controls was 50% and the RR=1.7 with 25% nonresponse among both cases and controls. What would the result (RR) have been without this nonresponse, if the exposure frequency was only half as high among the nonresponders as among the examined individuals in both cases and controls?

d. What problems may exist regarding the quality of the exposure information? How would this influence the relative risk?

e. What potential confounders (in addition to age and sex) should be taken into account?

20. A case-control study was conducted to investigate the effect of quitting cigarette smoking on the risk of developing a nonfatal myocardial infarction in men under the age of 55. During the period 1980–83 subjects were identified at 78 hospitals in the United States among men aged 20 to 54: those who had been hospitalized for their first myocardial infarction (potential cases) and a sample of those who had been hospitalized because of other diseases considered unrelated to smoking (potential controls). Those who had earlier cardiac diseases or angina pectoris were excluded. Of the remaining cases and controls 1,873 (87%) and 2,775 (93%), respectively, were examined regarding smoking habits and potential confounders. Compared with men who had never smoked, the relative risk was 2.9 (95% confidence interval 2.4–3.4) for "current smokers" (men who had smoked within the previous year), 2.0 (1.1–3.8) for men who gave up smoking 12 to 23 months previously, 1.1 (0.6–1.9) for men who gave up smoking 24 to 35 months previously, and close to 1 for men who gave up smoking 3 or more years previously.

a. What type of case-control study is this? How should the study base be defined if the hospitals in question did not have defined catchment areas (populations)?

b. Why were men with earlier cardiac diseases or angina pectoris excluded?

c. Can the choice of controls introduce a systematic error into the investigation even if the risk of developing the diseases of the controls is not influenced by smoking habits? How?

d. Information about smoking habits was collected by means of standardized interviews. Could misclassification with respect to smoking habits have influenced the results? In what way?

e. What potential confounders (in addition to age, earlier cardiac diseases, and earlier angina pectoris) should be taken into account?

11

Choice of Study Design

The choice of study design, like the choice of study base (Chapter 2) and choice of examination methods, is highly influenced by characteristics of the studied exposure and disease. As mentioned previously (Chapter 2), studies of the association between exposure and onset of disease are usually based on existing exposure conditions and on incident cases. If so, there is still a choice between different study designs where the study base is represented by a sample (case-control studies) or used in its entirety (cohort studies). In certain situations, however, exposure is assigned by the investigator with the purpose of improving validity (experimental studies). For some diseases it may be difficult or impossible to identify incident cases, and studies are then based on prevalent cases (cross-sectional studies). The subdivision of epidemiologic investigations is discussed in brief at the end of this chapter.

COHORT AND CASE-CONTROL STRATEGIES

When the investigation is planned, consideration should be given to the following:

1. *Incidence of the disease.* For a disease with a high incidence it may be natural to use a cohort design. For a disease with a low or moderate incidence, efficiency may be improved considerably if the study base is represented by a sample (case-control studies). In certain situations,

however, cohort studies may be made very efficient, e.g., by using information from existing registers. (See Chapters 4 and 6.)

2. *Exposure frequency.* The exposure frequency does not affect the choice between cohort and case-control design. In both types of studies, efficiency may be increased by choosing a study base with a high exposure frequency (up to 50% at RR=1). (See Chapters 4 and 6.)

3. *Induction period.* Contrary to some claims, the length of the induction time does not affect the choice between cohort and case-control design. If the induction time is long, results may be obtained in a substantially shorter time if retrospective or previously collected exposure information can be utilized (irrespective of the study design). (See Chapters 2, 4, 8, and 9.)

4. *Confounders.* The occurrence of confounders influences the validity of the investigation. The effect may be avoided through choice of the study base or controlled in the data analysis. (See Chapter 3.)

5. *Misclassification: exposure.* If the disease may be expected to influence the exposure information, this suggests the use of a type A case-control study or a cohort study. Sometimes one can solve the problem by examining the cases in a type B case-control study at an early stage (before the disease has influenced the exposure information). It has also been suggested that in a type C case-control study comparability with respect to the exposure information may be achieved by selecting controls in a suitable manner (See Chapters 3, 7–9.)

6 *Misclassification: disease.* If the exposure may be expected to affect the diagnosis of the disease, diagnostic criteria and examination routines should be chosen with this in mind, for example, by carrying out the diagnosis blind with respect to exposure. In certain situations exposed and unexposed individuals may be chosen so that comparability in terms of follow-up is achieved (See Chapter 3.)

7. *Cost: exposure information.* The higher the cost per individual of obtaining information about exposure condi-

tions (including relevant confounders), the greater the possibility of improving efficiency by means of case-control design (unless the incidence of the disease is so high that a large proportion of the individuals fall ill). Case-control studies of types B and C provide a higher efficiency than those of type A. It may be suitable to use an examination method that costs less per individual even if this means some increase in nondifferential misclassification. (See Chapters 4, 6–9.)

8. *Cost: diagnosis.* Identifying all cases of the disease that occur in the study base may require considerable resources. Sometimes these costs may be reduced by choosing another study base or other diagnostic criteria, or by utilizing information from, for example, various health and medical care registers. As in the case of exposure information, the cost must be weighed against the effect of any misclassification. (See Chapter 4.)

9. *Selection of controls.* If a type C case-control study involves difficulties in identifying a control group that reflects the occurrence of the exposure in the study base, the possibility of conducting a type B case-control study should be considered. This presupposes, as a rule, the choice of another study base and possibly another procedure for identifying the cases. (See Chapter 9.)

10. *Possibility of abstention.* In certain situations, on account of low validity or efficiency, one should refrain from conducting a planned investigation.

The study design should be chosen with due consideration of the validity and efficiency of the investigation. The cohort design is the primary choice for diseases with a high incidence or when the exposure information from a large study base is available at a low cost, e.g., from a register. The choice between prospective and retrospective exposure information in cohort studies is dependent on differences in quality and cost and on the length of the induction time. For diseases with a low or moderate incidence, the efficiency may be considerably improved if the study base is represented by a sample (case-control design). A type A case-control study does not, in principle, differ from the corresponding cohort study in terms of validity, but it may produce a higher level of efficiency (precision/cost). This applies particularly if the processing of raw data (e.g., analysis of specimens) involves appreciable costs. Use of a type B case-control study often leads to a considerably higher efficiency but assumes that the disease does not influence classification with regard to exposure. A type C case-control study may be an alternative if the study base is not available for random sampling, if comparability with regard to the quality of exposure information increases, or if the participation rate among the controls increases. This presupposes, however, that the controls reflect the exposure frequency in the study base.

OTHER DESIGN STRATEGIES

Three different strategies in study design will be discussed briefly here: experimental studies, cross-sectional studies ("prevalence studies"), and studies based on aggregated data ("ecologic studies").

Experimental Studies

Epidemiologic investigations are sometimes carried out with the aim of studying the effect of measures taken to change exposure conditions (intervention studies). Occasionally, exposure is assigned by the investigator with the aim of improving the validity of the study *(experimental studies)*, e.g., by randomly assigning exposure in the study population *(randomized experiments)*. The purpose of randomization is to control confounding. The advantage of this over other methods is that even the effect of unknown confounders can be controlled provided that the investigation is based on a sufficiently large number of individuals with randomization at an individual level. This does not prevent other methods of controlling confounding, e.g., restrictions in choice of the study base and stratification in the data analysis, from also being used (e.g., Byar et al. 1976; Campbell, Stanley 1966).

For ethical reasons, the intervention should be aimed at reducing disease occurrence (preventive measures), and participation in the study must not mean that some individuals must refrain from an alternative that is healthier according to current knowledge. Major randomized experiments have, for example, been conducted to study how antihypertensive drugs influence the risk of developing or dying from cardiovascular diseases, and also to study the effect of vaccination aimed at reducing the risk of contracting certain infectious diseases (e.g., Salk's vaccine and polio). However, practical problems may arise in relation to randomization at the individual level, e.g., if the intervention involves information aimed at influencing the individual's lifestyle at the same time as the individuals influence one another. When it is difficult or impossible to conduct randomization at the individual level (e.g., fluoridation of drinking water), various alternatives to a planned intervention may be considered (e.g., fluor tablets).

Randomized experiments may, as mentioned earlier (Chapter 2), be regarded as a variant of cohort studies. As in such studies, efficiency depends on exposure frequency, incidence of the disease, and the strength of the association. In experimental studies efficiency also depends on the intervention's power of penetration, i.e., the extent to which it changes exposure conditions. If, for example, the intervention consists of vaccination, the power of penetration may be high. If the intervention consists of information aimed at changing dietary and other habits in the long term, the power of penetration is, as a rule, considerably lower. This may reduce efficiency substantially compared with the corresponding cohort study (see Example 11.2). Low efficiency (high costs) means that experimental epidemiologic studies generally involve very common and/or serious diseases. Occasionally efficiency may be increased by conducting the intervention in such a way that the power of penetration is high or by choosing a study base in which the disease incidence is high (e.g. when the effect of preventive drug treatment on the risk of developing myocardial infarction is studied among individuals who have recovered from their first infarction). Some intervention studies are conducted, however, with an objective completely different from that of studying the association between exposure and disease, e.g., to study the power of penetration of the intervention.

For studying how a specific exposure influences the risk of falling ill, randomization affords a possibility of controlling the effect of unknown confounders, provided that such an investigation is conducted for ethical and practical reasons and with due regard to efficiency. In certain situations some form of placebo may be used, with the follow-up with respect to disease occurrence conducted blind, both for the participants and for the investigators (so-called double-blind studies).

> *Example 11.1:* A study was conducted to investigate how a high intake of vitamin C affects the risk of common cold. Of 300 healthy women between the ages of 50 and 69, half were selected at random for exposure (administration of certain doses of vitamin C in tablet form), and the others were given placebo tablets. The incidence of common cold was studied during a follow-up period of 6 months. The follow-up was carried out in such a way that neither the women studied nor the staff who examined them for disease occurrence knew which ones had received vitamin C or placebo, respectively.

> *Example 11.2:* In an investigation the intervention consisted of information about the importance of reducing fat consumption to a suitable level. One of the aims was to study how the incidence of colon cancer was affected, in order to reach conclusions about the association between fat consumption and colon cancer. The intervention was directed at half of the individuals in the study population; the remainder made up the comparison group. Diet interviews showed that 50% had a fat consumption above the level in question. A new examination showed that the intervention influenced knowledge in 40%, a quarter of whom reduced their fat consumption to the proposed level. A renewed examination a few years later

showed that only 20% of these individuals still had a low fat consumption. The proportion of the study population who showed a lasting reduction of fat intake from a raised ("exposed") to a suitable ("unexposed") level was therefore estimated at $0.5 \times 0.5 \times 0.4 \times 0.25 \times 0.2 = 0.005$. This represents the proportion of unexposed (by means of intervention) in the study population in the intervention study. In the corresponding cohort study (without intervention), the proportion of unexposed in the study population was 0.5. In other words, the intervention study requires about 100 times as great a study base as a cohort study to give a similar number of unexposed cases. For every 10 unexposed cases, the study base requirement in the intervention study is 4,100,000 person-years, and in the cohort study 41,000 person-years (at $RR = 1$; see Table 4.1). The corresponding case-control study would, for every 10 unexposed cases, comprise a total of (cases plus controls) 40 subjects (at $r=1$) or 100 subjects (at $r=4$). (See Table 6.1.)

Cross-Sectional Studies (Prevalence Studies)

Investigations of the association between exposure and onset of disease must in principle be based on comparisons of incidence (frequency of disease onset). In certain situations there is, however, only information about prevalent cases. This applies to, for example, studies of the association between exposure during pregnancy and malformations in the offspring. However, even when long-term chronic diseases with a low incidence are involved, it may be convenient to identify prevalent (rather than incident) cases. If on one sole occasion a health check or screening examination is carried out for the early detection of disease in a certain population, prevalent cases are identified. In investigations based on a comparison of prevalence there are, in addition to those discussed in Chapter 3, three other sources of systematic error:

1. The prevalence is due not only to the incidence of the disease but also to its duration (e.g., Ahlbom, Norell

1990). The association between exposure and disease prevalence is therefore influenced by a possible association between exposure and duration of the disease. This may introduce a systematic error in a study aimed at investigating how exposure influences the risk of falling ill. If the exposed individuals die or recover after a relatively short period of sickness, this results in an underestimation of the relative risk. In an investigation of congenital malformations, there may be reason to consider the possibility that malformed fetuses die and give rise to miscarriages or abortions. In an investigation of chronic diseases in adults, it is often impossible in practice to take into account any association between exposure and duration.

2. The disease may influence examination and classification with respect to exposure, since the individuals have already fallen ill when the examination is carried out. This is a potential source of error even in certain case-control studies (types B and C), but the exposure information is collected then, as a rule, a short time after the onset and diagnosis of the disease. In cross-sectional studies of diseases of long duration, the examination is often carried out long after the onset of the disease, which increases the risk of misclassification with respect to exposure during an etiologically relevant period. The result may be an over- or underestimation of the relative risk. In studies of congenital malformations, this source of error can be avoided if the exposure information is collected during pregnancy (Example 11.3).

3. The disease may influence the selection for the investigation (e.g., Kleinbaum et al. 1981). If individuals with the studied disease have a greater (or lesser) probability of being included in the study, this may introduce a systematic error (selection bias), with an over- or underestimation of the relative risk that is impossible to control in data analysis. In a study of congenital malformations, this can be avoided if the study comprises all children who are born during a certain period of time in a defined

population. But in an investigation based on, for example, the participants in a voluntary health checkup, this may be impossible to avoid (Example 11.4).

In cross-sectional studies it is not the frequency of onset of disease during a period of time (incidence) but the occurrence of disease at a point in time (prevalence) that is studied. The length of the follow-up period may be said to be zero. The study population consists of a cross-section of the population, where a subdivision into "closed" and "open" populations is no longer meaningful. Otherwise, conditions similar to those for cohort and case-control studies apply. This means that the study population may be represented in its entirety or by a sample. A sample of this kind may be made from the whole study population or possibly among those individuals who are not suffering from the studied disease [compare case-control studies, where the comparison is based on cumulative incidence (Chapter 6)].

In certain prevalence studies a cross-section of the "whole population" is used. This may be allowable for descriptive purposes, but for etiological studies this is considered an unsuitable study population in terms of the validity and efficiency of the investigation (Chapters 3 and 4). In addition, in some cross-sectional studies information about current exposure rather than exposure during an earlier, etiologically relevant period is collected. This means, however, that the induction period and possible change in exposure after the onset of the disease are ignored, which may introduce a systematic error.

Example 11.3: To investigate a possible association between the consumption of certain medicines during pregnancy and the occurrence of malformations in the newborn child, 5,000 pregnant mothers were interviewed about, among other things, drug consumption during pregnancy. Information about exposure and potential confounders (e.g., infections, tobacco, alcohol) was stored in the form of unprocessed data. Congenital malformations were established in 150 children. For every case four "controls" were selected at random from a list of the study population. Information from cases and controls was encoded blind.

Example 11.4: All women of certain ages resident in a certain area were offered a mammography examination for early detection of breast cancer. During the previous year an investigation had detected an increased risk of breast cancer among women with a long-term consumption of contraceptive pills, which attracted attention in the media. There was a discussion about the possibility of studying the association between contraceptive pills and the occurrence of breast cancer among those examined in the mammography checkup. However, this may represent an unsuitable study population on account of the risk of selection bias. Assume, for example, that women who themselves have detected suspect abnormalities in their breasts (some of whom have breast cancer) are more inclined to schedule health checkups, especially if they have used contraceptive pills. Such a selection would result in an overestimation of the proportion of sick people among the exposed individuals, compared with the proportion of sick among the unexposed.

Aggregated Data (Ecologic Studies)

Occasionally one sees figures that show a striking covariance between, for example, average fat consumption per capita in different countries and mortality from some form of cancer or cardiovascular disease. Such a study differs in one important respect from all the investigations discussed previously: The observations do not refer to individuals but to average "exposure" and mortality in different populations (aggregates). This influences the interpretation of the results. Data provide, for example, no information about the distribution of the exposure in the population or about the extent to which the individuals who died from the disease were exposed. Above all, however, there is generally a lack of information necessary to control the effect of potential confounders. Nevertheless, a possible covariance may help to generate hypotheses and stimulate epidemiologic studies of the kind discussed earlier. The costs may, moreover, be low if the information can be obtained from official publications (e.g., sales, mortality, and population statistics). Different methods have been proposed to reduce the importance of certain sources of error in so-called ecologic studies (e.g., Morgenstern 1982).

SUBDIVISION OF EPIDEMIOLOGIC STUDIES

Epidemiologic investigations are, by tradition, usually subdivided into cohort studies and case-control studies. (This applies to studies of the association between exposure and onset of disease, with information at the individual level.) As is apparent from Chapter 6, cohort and case-control studies differ with regard to the manner in which the study base is represented. In this respect, case-control studies of types A and B and case-control studies of type C also differ. The subdivision of epidemiologic investigations that has been used here (Chapters 2, 6–9) is based on the representation of the study base and the time of the exposure information. Whether the exposure information is collected primarily before or after the onset of disease is decisive in terms of both validity and efficiency (Chapters 3 and 8). In type A case-control studies information about exposure conditions is collected before the onset of disease, but in type B and C case-control studies this information is collected after the onset of the disease. See Table 11.1.

TABLE 11.1. *Subdivision of case-control studies according to representation of the study base and time of collecting the exposure information*

Type of study	Study base representation	Time of collecting exposure information
Case-control study A	Random sample	Before disease onset
Case-control study B	Random sample	After disease onset
Case-control study C	Other sample	After disease onset

The representation of the study base and the time of the exposure information may affect the validity and efficiency of the investigation to a high degree (Chapters 3–4, 6–9). To avoid systematic errors, it is necessary in cohort studies to take into account any possible confounding and misclassification with respect to exposure and disease. For type A case-control studies the same conditions regarding systematic errors apply in principle. In type B case-control studies there is, in addition, the possibility that the disease may affect classification with respect to exposure. In type C case-control studies there is yet another potential source of error: The choice of controls may introduce a systematic error. As a rule, the efficiency of the investigation increases considerably if the study base is represented by a sample (case-control studies), particularly if the exposure information can be collected after the onset of the disease (types B and C). The extent of the advantage gained depends on the difference between the size of the study base and the size of the sample (number of controls) and on the cost per individual. The efficiency increases most when the cost is high and the disease incidence is low.

In addition to the designs described here, it is possible under certain conditions to consider cohort studies in which the exposure information is collected after the onset of the disease. (The study population should, even in this situation, be defined before the start of the follow-up period.) In case-control studies in which primary information on exposure is collected before the onset of the disease, there occasionally is reason to let the study base be represented by something other than a random sample.

Within the framework of an investigation, use is sometimes made of more than one alternative regarding the representation of the study base, for example, by means of selecting both hospital controls and a random sample of the study base (type B+C case-control studies). Occasionally more than one alternative is used with regard to the time for exposure information; for example, simpler (cheaper) exposure information collected before the onset of the disease may be used along with more detailed (and costly) exposure information collected after the onset of the disease (type A+B case-control studies).

Epidemiologic investigations may, of course, also differ in other respects. In the subdivision of investigations, account is sometimes taken of whether previously collected information regarding exposure and disease was used ("retrospective cohort studies") or of the sampling method used ("matched case-control studies"). Other distinctions are based on, for example, the type of study population, open or closed ("nested case-control study" = a case-control study with a closed study population); the method of obtaining exposure information (interview/questionnaire, observation, measurement); and diagnosis (e.g., blind in relation to exposure). Intervention studies, particularly randomized experiments, are as a rule regarded as a special type of epidemiologic study. Even though it may be fruitful to subdivide epidemiologic investigations on the basis of, for example, the representation of the study base and the time of exposure information, all studies are based on the principle that applies to cohort studies: comparison of the occurrence of disease among different sections of the study base that differ in terms of exposure.

12

Interpretation of Results

The results of the investigation are generally reported in the form of relative risks with, for example, 95% confidence intervals. The relative risk provides information about the direction and strength of the observed association, and the confidence interval provides information about the precision of the investigation (Chapter 4). The report should, in addition, contain information that enables the reader to evaluate different sources of systematic errors. The interpretation of the results is naturally dependent to a high degree on the accuracy of the investigation. There is no reason to regard case-control studies in general as less accurate or credible than cohort studies. On the other hand, bearing in mind the results and the design of the study, there is reason to give careful consideration to different potential sources of error (Chapters 2–4, 6–9).

When the results show an association between exposure and disease:

1. Is it likely that the observed association can be explained by *random error?* The confidence interval reflects the precision of the investigation.
2. Are there potential *confounders* that can explain the observed association? What confounders have been taken into account in the investigation? May other confounders (which ones?) have influenced the result? In what direction?
3. May *misclassification* explain the observed association?

a. Could the occurrence of exposure have influenced the identification of the cases? How? In what direction would this influence the result?
b. Could the disease have influenced the classification with respect to exposure? How? In what direction would this influence the result? (This applies to type B and C case-control studies.) Nondifferential misclassification is not of interest here, apart from the fact that it may contribute to an underestimation of the strength of the association.

When the results do not show any association between exposure and disease:

1. Is the *random error* so great (the confidence interval so wide) that the result is compatible with an appreciable association between exposure and disease? If this is the case, the result must be interpreted to mean that the investigation is not sufficiently informative.
2. Are there potential *confounders* that might conceal an association? What confounders have been taken into account in the investigation? May other confounders (which ones?) have influenced the result? In what direction?
3. May *misclassification* conceal an association? Here, the same questions apply as when an association is indicated. In addition, consideration must be given to any nondifferential misclassification (with respect to exposure or disease) that may contribute to the concealment of an association.

Irrespective of what the results show, consideration should be given to how *nonparticipation* may have influenced the result of the investigation (e.g., Chapter 5, Exercise 3). This involves subjects lost to the follow-up and classification with respect to disease [irrespective of the study design (Chapter 3)] and subjects lost to the examination and classification with respect to exposure among cases and controls [in type B and C case-control studies (Chapter 8). If the investigation is a type C case-control study, the following questions also apply:

Can the *choice of control group* have introduced a systematic error into the investigation? In which direction may this have influenced the result? (See Chapter 9.) In investigations where the comparison is based on prevalence (cross-sectional studies), there are further potential sources of error. (See Chapter 11.)

Many apparently contradictory results from different epidemiologic investigations can probably be ascribed to "negative findings" due to nondifferential misclassification and low precision. The latter may to a certain extent be ascribed to the previous practice of reporting results of hypothesis testing rather than using a confidence interval. Studies that did not show a "significant" association were then often judged as "negative" even if the precision was low, i.e., where a confidence interval would contain appreciable associations (e.g., Walker 1986a). Confounding and differential misclassification may explain both false "positive" and false "negative" findings. The same applies to the choice of controls in type C case-control studies.

There are many examples of overly far-reaching conclusions drawn from results of individual epidemiologic investigations. There may be several reasons for this. In scientific literature greater cautiousness is often exercised in the interpretation of results than that reflected in the general debate. Individual researchers occasionally, however, have an interest in using "striking" findings to spread information about their own research. In addition, there is an interest on the part of the media in spreading news, perhaps in the form of "remarkable" or "frightening" results of individual investigations. There is also, quite naturally, concern on the part of the general public about real or experienced health risks and, consequently, a great susceptibility to "alarming reports." At the same time, information and knowledge about different problems of methodology and sources of error are greatly limited as a rule. Expectations are often overly great regarding the "value as evidence" of results of individual investigations.

There are also examples of general reservations in the interpretation of results of epidemiologic investigations. It is occasionally said that epidemiologic studies can establish only statistical associations. It is unclear what is meant by this. A literal interpretation is not feasible since "statistical associations" are also established in animal experiments, clinical investigations, and other empirical research. Perhaps the underlying intent is that it is possible in epidemiology to study only covariance between exposure and disease. This is a misconception, since the central role of control of confounding in epidemiology is disregarded (Chapter 3). The question of whether the methods used to control confounding (restriction, standardization, randomization, etc.) are satisfactory is a matter that must be assessed for the individual investigation.

CAUSALITY

When is it possible to conclude that an observed association represents a causal association? This question is as old as research into the etiology of diseases, and the history of medicine contains a number of suggested criteria. Among the best known are the Henle-Koch postulates, which, however, refer solely to the association between infecting agents and infectious diseases (e.g., Evans 1978). In the field of epidemiology, more general criteria have been proposed by Hill (Hill 1965) and others. These must not be taken as definitive, but they may nevertheless provide some guidance in an assessment. In this connection, the result of the individual investigation must be viewed in relation to previous knowledge that is relevant to the studied association. In making the assessment, account should be taken of the following:

1. *The accuracy of the investigation.* The importance of random and systematic errors is discussed in brief at the beginning of this chapter. See also Chapters 3–4 and 6–9.
2. *The statistical properties of the association.* Credibility is often considered to increase with the strength of the association (deviation from RR=1) and with so-called dose-response patterns (stronger associations at higher exposure

levels). However, it should be noted that a causal association may very well exist even if the association is not strong, and that dose-response patterns do not exclude confounding.

3. *Results of other investigations.* Credibility increases if several investigations with different material (study base) and methods (design, examination methods) show similar results. It is not sufficient, however, to compare the number of "positive" and "negative" studies. Every investigation must be assessed in terms of accuracy. Apparent contradictions between results may be due to effect modification (Chapter 1), i.e., the exposure may have different effects in different sections of the population. (See the following discussion of generalizability.)

4. *Biological credibility.* In the assessment of the results of the investigation, account should naturally be taken of what is known in other respects about the biological effects of the exposure. This may apply, for example, to results of mutagenicity tests or animal experiments. There are, however, several examples of epidemiologic studies that found an association between exposure and disease long before the results received support from other research (e.g., Terris 1964).

The question of how to interpret associations that fulfill criteria 1 and 3 (and possibly 2) but not 4 is of particular interest. If it was not possible in the investigation to take into account unknown confounders by random assignment of exposure, the possible existence of a previously unknown etiological factor covariant with the studied exposure should be carefully considered. The observed association may be a step on the way toward identifying such a factor and, as a result, achieving increased knowledge about the etiology of the disease. Another possibility is, of course, that there is a causal association, or that sufficiently exacting demands were not established in relation to the first three criteria, and no association exists. The relationship between covariance and causal association, as well as the use of causal models in epidemiology, is discussed elsewhere (Ahlbom, Norell 1990).

For a study with no random or systematic error, the relative risk would represent the true causal association (if any) in the study base. Any differences between such studies would reflect true differences in effect due to effect modification. Other criteria would not be needed. However, the possibility of random or systematic error (such as unrecognized confounding or misclassification) can never be excluded in empirical science (including epidemiology). As Lakatos (1984) puts it, "Very few philosophers or scientists still think that scientific knowledge is, or can be, proven knowledge."

In spite of this basic uncertainty, there is often a need to make decisions on the basis of scientific information. For instance, decisions on the implementation of prevention programs in public health may be based on reports from epidemiologic research. In this context, "criteria" such as those mentioned previously have been proposed as an aid for judging whether an observed association is causal. It has been argued, however, that progress in scientific knowledge is made only by falsification (Popper 1963), and that epidemiologic research should involve the search for error and alternative explanations rather than looking for "causal criteria" (e.g., Lanes 1988a,b).

GENERALIZABILITY

An important question is the *generalizability* of the results, i.e., to what extent they apply outside the study base. If, for example, the association between smoking and lung cancer that has been established in several epidemiologic studies applied only to the individuals included in these investigations, the results would be of very limited value. Using knowledge about the association between exposure and disease with prevention in mind involves consideration of the possibilities of generalizing for the future. The study base can never be selected as a random sample of such future populations, and the generalizability of the results is consequently not a question of statistical inference. It is instead a question of appraisal based on knowledge about the biological and other conditions under which the association was observed.

The question of the extent to which the results can be generalized outside the study base is, of course, meaningful only if the results apply to the study base itself. Any generalization presupposes that the results are accurate. One should therefore avoid trying to "increase the generalizability" at the expense of accuracy.

The generalizability of the results is, as a rule, a considerably lesser problem in epidemiology than in animal experiments in which there is a wish to draw conclusions about the association between exposure and disease in human beings. (In general, the differences between human beings are considerably smaller than the differences between human beings and animals.) Instead, the validity of the results is a fundamental question for epidemiologic investigations. This does not mean that one should not consider the generalizability of the results carefully. An association (exposure-disease) may exist in one section of the population (e.g., among women of fertile ages) but not in others (e.g., among men and older women). Generalizability is limited if the effect of the exposure differs in different sections of the population (effect modification—see Chapter 1). As for reaching a decision on the generalizability of the results, one should therefore consider what modifying factors may influence the observed association (e.g., age, sex, or the occurrence of certain other exposures that influence the risk of developing the studied disease). If such factors are expected to influence (modify) the observed association, there may be reason to investigate the association in different sections of the population.

13

Tables

TABLE 13.1 *Nondifferential misclassification with respect to exposure: Estimated relative risk for different exposure frequencies, true relative risk (RR) levels, sensitivities, and specificities. [Premise: The probability of being classified as exposed is at least as great among the exposed as among the unexposed, i.e., (sensitivity + specificity) ≥ 1.]*

		Sensitivity				
Specificity:		1.0	0.8	0.6	0.4	0.2
Estimated relative risk at exposure frequency of 50%						
RR = 4	1.0	4.00	2.67	2.15	1.88	1.71
	0.8	3.50	2.13	1.63	1.31	1.00
	0.6	3.14	1.71	1.27	1.00	
	0.4	2.88	1.36	1.00		
	0.2	2.67	1.00			
RR = 2	1.0	2.00	1.71	1.56	1.45	1.38
	0.8	1.83	1.50	1.31	1.17	1.00
	0.6	1.71	1.33	1.14	1.00	
	0.4	1.63	1.18	1.00		
	0.2	1.56	1.00			
RR = 0.5	1.0	0.50	0.55	0.58	0.62	0.64
	0.8	0.58	0.67	0.75	0.85	1.00
	0.6	0.64	0.76	0.88	1.00	
	0.4	0.69	0.86	1.00		
	0.2	0.72	1.00			
Estimated relative risk at exposure frequency of 10%						
RR = 4	1.0	4.00	3.76	3.55	3.37	3.21
	0.8	2.07	1.78	1.51	1.26	1.00
	0.6	1.65	1.40	1.18	1.00	
	0.4	1.47	1.20	1.00		
	0.2	1.37	1.00			

TABLE 13.1 *Continued.*

	Specificity:	Sensitivity				
		1.0	0.8	0.6	0.4	0.2
RR=2	1.0	2.00	1.96	1.92	1.88	1.85
	0.8	1.36	1.27	1.19	1.10	1.00
	0.6	1.22	1.14	1.07	1.00	
	0.4	1.16	1.07	1.00		
	0.2	1.12	1.00			
RR=0.5	1.0	0.50	0.51	0.51	0.52	0.52
	0.8	0.82	0.86	0.90	0.95	1.00
	0.6	0.89	0.93	0.96	1.00	
	0.4	0.92	0.96	1.00		
	0.2	0.94	1.00			
Estimated relative risk at exposure frequency of 2%						
RR=4	1.0	4.00	3.95	3.91	3.86	3.82
	0.8	1.28	1.21	1.14	1.07	1.00
	0.6	1.15	1.10	1.05	1.00	
	0.4	1.10	1.05	1.00		
	0.2	1.07	1.00			
RR=2	1.0	2.00	1.99	1.98	1.98	1.97
	0.8	1.09	1.07	1.05	1.02	1.00
	0.6	1.05	1.03	1.02	1.00	
	0.4	1.03	1.02	1.00		
	0.2	1.02	1.00			
RR=0.5	1.0	0.50	0.50	0.50	0.50	0.50
	0.8	0.95	0.96	0.98	0.99	1.00
	0.6	0.98	0.98	0.99	1.00	
	0.4	0.98	0.99	1.00		
	0.2	0.99	1.00			

Sensitivity: (number of exposed who are classified as exposed)/(number of exposed), i.e., the probability of an exposed individual being classified as exposed.

Specificity: (number of unexposed who are classified as unexposed)/(number of unexposed), i.e., the probability of an unexposed individual being classified as unexposed.

(See Chapter 3 for more information.)

TABLE 13.2 *Power, i.e., the probability of establishing (as statistically significant, p < 0.05, two-tailed test) an association of a certain strength (RR) at different exposure frequencies and study sizes (number of cases).*

		Number of cases (exposed + unexposed)				
	Exp.· (%):	50	100	200	400	800
Cohort study with large study base (0.3 million person-years)						
RR = 8	50	1.00	1.00	1.00	1.00	1.00
	25	1.00	1.00	1.00	1.00	1.00
	10	1.00	1.00	1.00	1.00	1.00
	5	0.99	1.00	1.00	1.00	1.00
	2	0.92	0.99	1.00	1.00	1.00
	1	0.69	0.94	1.00	1.00	1.00
RR = 4	50	0.98	1.00	1.00	1.00	1.00
	25	0.99	1.00	1.00	1.00	1.00
	10	0.95	1.00	1.00	1.00	1.00
	5	0.83	0.97	1.00	1.00	1.00
	2	0.57	0.81	0.97	1.00	1.00
	1	0.38	0.59	0.83	0.98	1.00
RR = 2	50	0.60	0.90	1.00	1.00	1.00
	25	0.61	0.88	0.99	1.00	1.00
	10	0.42	0.68	0.92	1.00	1.00
	5	0.27	0.47	0.73	0.95	1.00
	2	0.14	0.25	0.43	0.69	0.93
	1	0.08	0.15	0.26	0.44	0.71
RR = 0.5	50	0.60	0.90	1.00	1.00	1.00
	25	0.33	0.69	0.96	1.00	1.00
	10	0.08	0.14	0.59	0.94	1.00
	5	0.02	0.07	0.24	0.61	0.95
	2	0.00	0.01	0.05	0.17	0.50
	1	0.00	0.00	0.01	0.05	0.18
Case-control study (number of controls/number of cases = 4)						
RR = 8	50	1.00	1.00	1.00	1.00	1.00
	25	1.00	1.00	1.00	1.00	1.00
	10	1.00	1.00	1.00	1.00	1.00
	5	0.98	1.00	1.00	1.00	1.00
	2	0.81	0.97	1.00	1.00	1.00
	1	0.56	0.83	0.98	1.00	1.00
RR = 4	50	0.98	1.00	1.00	1.00	1.00
	25	0.98	1.00	1.00	1.00	1.00
	10	0.90	1.00	1.00	1.00	1.00
	5	0.70	0.94	1.00	1.00	1.00
	2	0.39	0.66	0.91	0.99	1.00
	1	0.21	0.41	0.68	0.91	1.00

TABLE 13.2 *Continued.*

	Exp.' (%):	Number of cases (exposed + unexposed)				
		50	100	200	400	800
RR=2	50	0.50	0.83	0.99	1.00	1.00
	25	0.49	0.80	0.98	1.00	1.00
	10	0.30	0.55	0.84	0.99	1.00
	5	0.18	0.34	0.60	0.87	0.99
	2	0.08	0.16	0.30	0.54	0.82
	1	0.04	0.09	0.17	0.31	0.55
RR=0.5	50	0.50	0.83	0.99	1.00	1.00
	25	0.27	0.59	0.91	1.00	1.00
	10	0.08	0.21	0.50	0.86	0.99
	5	0.03	0.08	0.21	0.50	0.87
	2	0.01	0.02	0.05	0.15	0.39
	1	0.00	0.01	0.02	0.05	0.15

Case-control study (number of controls/number of cases = 1)

		50	100	200	400	800
RR=8	50	0.99	1.00	1.00	1.00	1.00
	25	1.00	1.00	1.00	1.00	1.00
	10	0.98	1.00	1.00	1.00	1.00
	5	0.86	1.00	1.00	1.00	1.00
	2	0.45	0.83	0.99	1.00	1.00
	1	0.19	0.48	0.85	0.99	1.00
RR=4	50	0.85	0.99	1.00	1.00	1.00
	25	0.88	1.00	1.00	1.00	1.00
	10	0.65	0.94	1.00	1.00	1.00
	5	0.38	0.73	0.97	1.00	1.00
	2	0.13	0.32	0.66	0.94	1.00
	1	0.05	0.14	0.34	0.68	0.95
RR=2	50	0.32	0.61	0.91	1.00	1.00
	25	0.28	0.56	0.88	0.99	1.00
	10	0.14	0.31	0.60	0.90	1.00
	5	0.07	0.16	0.34	0.64	0.92
	2	0.02	0.06	0.13	0.29	0.56
	1	0.01	0.02	0.06	0.13	0.29
RR=0.5	50	0.32	0.61	0.91	1.00	1.00
	25	0.19	0.41	0.73	0.96	1.00
	10	0.07	0.17	0.36	0.67	0.94
	5	0.03	0.08	0.17	0.37	0.68
	2	0.01	0.02	0.06	0.14	0.29
	1	0.00	0.01	0.02	0.06	0.14

'Exp., exposure frequency in the study base for cohort study, or for case-control study among controls.

(For discussion, see Chapter 4.)

14

Glossary

Accuracy Absence of systematic and random error.

Bias See *systematic error.*

Case An episode or onset of disease in a subject. An individual who falls sick several times during the follow-up period represents one sick individual (see *cumulative incidence*) but several cases (unless the study is limited to, for example, the first onset of disease) (see *incidence rate*).

Case-control study (case-referent study) Investigation of the association between exposure and onset of disease in which use is made of exposure information from a sample of the study base. (Compare *cohort study.*)

Closed population (fixed population, cohort) A population in which the same individuals are followed from the start of the follow-up period until its end (or until their deaths). (Compare *open population.*)

Cohort study (follow-up study) Investigation of the association between exposure and onset of disease where use is made of exposure information from the whole study base. (The term *cohort study* is sometimes used for such studies only if the study population is closed.) (Compare *case-control study.*)

Confounder (confounding factor) A factor that is covariant with the studied exposure in the study base and influences the risk of developing the studied disease (over and above what is occasioned by any association between exposure and disease).

Confounding   The systematic error that is introduced by a confounder.

Cumulative incidence   The number of individuals who fall sick during the follow-up period divided by the number of individuals free from the disease at the beginning of the period (in a closed population).

Dose-response pattern   Increasing strength of the association (deviation from RR=1) with increasing exposure level.

Effect modification   Change in the impact of a certain exposure on disease incidence brought about by another (modifying) factor.

Efficiency (cost-efficiency)   Precision in relation to the cost of a study. (Compare *size-efficiency,* precision in relation to the size of a study.)

Epidemiology   The study of disease occurrence.

Experiment   A study where the exposure is assigned (manipulated) by the investigator with the aim of improving the validity of the study, e.g., by means of random assignment of exposure in the study population (randomized experiment).

Exposure   Characteristic or event that might influence the frequency of disease onset. (The term *exposure* is sometimes limited to such characteristics of the environment.)

Follow-up period   Period of time during which the study population is observed with respect to disease onset.

Generalizability (external validity)   Applicability (of the result) outside the study base.

Incidence   Frequency of disease onset (measures: incidence rate, cumulative incidence). (Compare *prevalence.*)

Incidence rate (incidence density)   Number of new cases of the disease divided by the amount of person-time in (the corresponding part of) the study base.

Induction period   Time from exposure to effect (onset of disease). (Compare *latent period.*)

Latent period   Time from disease onset to diagnosis.

Matching   Selection of a group that is similar to a given group in the distribution of one or more variables.

Matching of controls to cases   Selection of controls (i.e., a sample of the study base or study population) that are similar to the cases in the distribution of one or more variables (e.g., age, sex).

Matching of unexposed to exposed Selection of unexposed individuals that are similar to the exposed in the distribution of one or more variables (e.g., age, sex).

Misclassification Classifying individuals in the wrong category with respect to, for example, exposure or disease. (See *sensitivity, specificity, nondifferential misclassification.*)

Nondifferential misclassification (1) With respect to disease: Misclassification with the same sensitivity and specificity for the exposed and the unexposed. (2) With respect to exposure: Misclassification with the same sensitivity and specificity for cases and noncases.

Open population (dynamic population) A population in and out of which individuals move during the follow-up period (e.g., the population in a town with people moving in and out). (Compare *closed population.*)

Person-time (person-years) Sum of the number of time units (years) of follow-up for each subject (for example in the study base or a portion thereof, e.g., the exposed).

Population Group of individuals, for example, the study population (i.e., the individuals included in the investigation). (See *closed population, open population.*)

Precision Absence of random error.

Prevalence Number of sick individuals divided by the total number of individuals at a certain point in time.

Random error Difference between an empirical value and the average empirical value (in an infinite number of studies using the same methodology). (Compare *systematic error.*)

Randomized experiment See *experiment.*

Relative risk (RR) Disease incidence among exposed divided by the disease incidence among unexposed (with disease incidence expressed as incidence rate or cumulative incidence). (Compare *crude relative risk,* where account is not taken of confounders in the data analysis, and *standardized relative risk,* where account is taken in the data analysis

of one or more confounders by means of standardization.)
(See also *standardized mortality (morbidity) ratio.*)

Risk factor Cause of disease (sometimes also used as a synonym for *risk indicator*).

Risk indicator Characteristic or event that occurs before and is covariant with the occurrence of disease (i.e., indicates an increased or decreased risk of falling ill).

Sensitivity (1) In classification with respect to disease: Number of sick individuals who are classified as sick divided by the number of sick individuals (i.e., the probability of a sick individual being classified as sick). (2) In classification with respect to exposure: Number of exposed individuals who are classified as exposed divided by the number of exposed individuals (i.e., the probability of an exposed individual being classified as exposed). (Compare *specificity.*)

Specificity (1) In classification with respect to disease: Number of healthy individuals who are classified as healthy divided by the number of healthy individuals (i.e., the probability of a healthy individual being classified as healthy, in terms of the studied disease). (2) In classification with respect to exposure: Number of unexposed individuals who are classified as unexposed divided by the number of unexposed individuals (i.e., the probability of an unexposed individual being classified as unexposed). (Compare *sensitivity.*)

Standardized mortality (morbidity) ratio (SMR) Observed number of deaths (cases) divided by the expected number of deaths (cases). Corresponds to the death rate (incidence rate) among the exposed divided by death rate (incidence rate) among the unexposed, where in the data analysis account has been taken of one or more confounders by means of so-called indirect standardization (i.e., using weights proportional to the distribution of the exposed). (Compare *relative risk.*)

Stratification Subdivision into categories (strata) with respect to one or more variables (e.g., age groups). (See *stratified analysis* and *stratified sampling.*)

Stratified analysis Data analysis where the association is analyzed after stratification based on one or more variables (e.g., to control confounding from such variables). (See *stratification.*)

Stratified sampling Sampling with different factions among strata in the population. (See *stratification.*)

Study base The "person-time-experience" that is studied with respect to disease occurrence, i.e., the study population during the follow-up period.

Study population See *population.*

Systematic error (bias) The difference between the true value and the average empirical value (in an infinite number of studies using the same methodology). (Compare *random error.*)

Validity (internal validity) Absence of systematic error.

15

Answers to Exercises

1. a.
$$RR = \frac{97/1,626}{71/1,840} = 1.5$$

 b.
$$RR = \frac{19/628}{46/1,524} = 1.0$$

 c.
$$RR = \frac{78/998}{25/316} = 1.0$$

 d. No.

 e. Cumulative incidence.

 f. Some underestimation of a, but b and c not affected.

 g. Some underestimation of a, b, and c.

2. a. Exposure frequency=5% instead of 10%, i.e., a marked underestimation of the exposure frequency.

 b. Relative risk=1.9 instead of 2.0, i.e., a small underestimation of the strength of the association (see Tables section). The calculation may be done in the following manner: Assume that k is the number of subjects in the study population, of whom 10% were exposed ($0.1 \times k$) and 90% were unexposed ($0.9 \times k$):

	Exposed	Unexposed
Cases	a	b
Study population	$0.1 \times k$	$0.9 \times k$

$$RR = \frac{a/(0.1 \times k)}{b/(0.9 \times k)} = 2 \qquad b = 4.5 \times a$$

With nondifferential misclassification, sensitivity= 0.5, and specificity=1.0:

	"Exposed"	"Unexposed"
Cases	$0.5 \times a$	$4.5 \times a + 0.5 \times a$
Study population	$0.5 \times 0.1 \times k$	$0.9 \times k + 0.5 \times 0.1 \times k$

$$RR = \frac{0.5a/(0.5 \times 0.1 \times k)}{(4.5a + 0.5a)/(0.9k + 0.5 \times 0.1 \times k)} = 1.9$$

3.

	Exposed	Unexposed
Cases	a	b
Study base	C	D

Nonparticipation: 2% of the exposed ($0.02C$), 15% of the unexposed ($0.15D$). The risk of developing disease in those who did not participate in the follow-up was twice as high, i.e., $2(a/C)$ among the exposed and $2(b/D)$ among the unexposed. Number of cases in those who did not participate:

$$\text{Exposed} = 2(0.02a) = 0.04a$$
$$\text{Unexposed} = 2(0.15b) = 0.30b$$

Results based on participants:

	Exposed	Unexposed
Cases	$a - 0.04a$	$b - 0.30b$
Study base	$C - 0.02C$	$D - 0.15D$

$$RR = \frac{(a-0.04a)(D-0.15D)}{(b-0.30b)(C-0.02C)} = \frac{0.96 \times 0.85}{0.70 \times 0.98} \times \frac{aD}{bC}$$

But aD/bC = 1; hence, *RR = 1.2* (instead of RR = 1.0).

4. RR=1 and exposure frequency=25%, i.e., for every exposed case there are four cases. $I=2 \times 10^{-3}$ per year, i.e., two cases per 1,000 person-years: For every case there are 500 person-years. Hence, 30 exposed cases require 4×30=120 cases and 120×500=*60,000 person-years.*

5. Approximately 10% (or higher, if one takes into account possible nonparticipation and nondifferential misclassification).

6. a. The study population was infants born July 1, 1977–June 30, 1982 to mothers who had been members of the Seattle GHC for at least 280 days. The length of the follow-up period was not specified, but the disease is diagnosed within a few months after birth.

   b. For the women who became members during pregnancy, information was lacking about prescriptions filled during the relevant period.

   c. The drug (Bendectin) exposure of the fetus (theoretically) and prescriptions filled by the mother during pregnancy (empirically). If, for example, some mothers filled prescriptions but did not consume Bendectin during pregnancy (or vice versa), this would result in a misclassification with respect to exposure. The expected effect is an underestimation of the strength of the association (RR→1). A survey showed that over 95% of female members filled their prescriptions at GHC pharmacies.

   d. A subdivision was made based on the number of

prescriptions filled (the vast majority were for a 28-day supply):

Number of orders	RR (95% confidence interval)
1	1.24 (0.36-4.35)
2–4	2.30 (0.85-6.27)
5+	7.59 (4.95-11.64)

A subdivision of exposure based on different periods of time during pregnancy would also be of interest (see Exercise 16, Chapter 10).

These subdivisions provide an opportunity to study so-called dose-response patterns (stronger association at higher exposure levels) and the time relation between effective exposure and organ development in the fetus. The primary limitation in a subdivision into several exposure categories is lower precision (wider confidence intervals).

e. All cases of the disease that occur in the study base should be identified. Members of the GHC were treated, with few exceptions, at certain hospitals. The disease is diagnosed (and operated on) as a rule within a few months after the child's birth. To check that the identified cases fulfilled the diagnostic criteria, their records were scrutinized. This was carried out blind, i.e., without knowledge of the exposure conditions. In all 26 cases that fulfilled the diagnostic criteria, the diagnosis was confirmed during the operation.

f. By means of comparison with women who received other treatment for nausea during pregnancy. This could not be carried out, however, in the current study: Over 90% of the women who were treated for nausea during pregnancy were given Bendectin.

g. The mother's age and calendar time were considered but found not to be important confounders (controlled by stratification in the data analysis). Other potential confounders discussed included smoking and other drugs consumed during pregnancy, length of gestation, birth order, and sex of the infant (see Exercise 16, Chapter 10).

(Aselton P et al: Pyloric stenosis and maternal Bendectin exposure. *Am J Epidemiol* 1984;120:251-6.)

7. a. All gainfully employed male workers aged 20 to 64 in the Swedish National Census of 1960 followed up over a 19-year period (1961–79).

   b. Exposure to wood dust in the respiratory tract (theoretical) and employment as a furniture worker according to the National Census 60 (empirical).

   c. The advantage is that existing exposure information (information on occupation in the 1960 census) may be used at a low cost. The study can therefore be based on a large number of individuals (at a reasonable cost), which produces a relatively high precision. Despite this, only 11 cases of adenocarcinoma were observed in the nasal cavity among 8,141 furniture workers during the course of 19 years. If the study base comprises substantially fewer exposed individuals and/or shorter follow-up periods, the precision would be low.

   The disadvantage is that information is lacking about the extent to which individual persons were exposed to wood dust in the respiratory tracts. A number of furniture workers may have been practically unexposed, and a number of the other ("unexposed") employed workers may have been exposed to wood dust (through working as furniture workers before or after 1960, in other occupations, or in their leisure time). This would result in an underestimation of the strength of the association (RR→1). The lack of information about specific exposure also means that a subdivision into different exposure levels (low exposed, high exposed) is not possible, and that the effect of wood dust cannot be distinguished from a possible effect of other exposures in the same work environment (see f).

d. If a large proportion of the identified furniture workers in the national census were not working in this occupation 10 years earlier, this would mean an underestimation of the strength of the association (RR→1) during the first part of the follow-up period.

e. Sex and occupational class by means of restrictions in the choice of the study base (the investigation covered only male workers). Age and area of residence (county) by means of stratification in the data analysis.

f. Smoking and any other factors that may conceivably be covariant with the exposure and influence the risk of developing malignant tumors in the respiratory tract. If smoking was more common among furniture workers than among other workers one would, however, expect an overrisk of lung cancer (but RR=0.9; 95% confidence interval 0.7–1.1). The effect of certain other exposures in the same work environment (e.g., paint, varnish, solvents) may in principle be studied in a corresponding investigation of, for example, painters.

g. An underdiagnosis of the same magnitude among furniture workers and other workers (nondifferential misclassification) would not influence RR (but would produce fewer observed cases and, consequently, wider confidence intervals). The corresponding overdiagnosis would produce an underestimation of the strength of the association (RR→1). A misclassification (under- or overdiagnosis) influenced by, for example, age or area of residence (county) would give an underestimation of the strength of the association (RR→1) after stratification for age and county, respectively, in the data analysis. A misclassification influenced by the exposure (or by a factor not been treated as a confounder in the investigation) might produce an over- or underestimation of RR.

(Gerhardsson MR et al: Respiratory cancers in furniture workers. *Br J Ind Med* 1985;42:403-5.)

8. a. The study base was a sample of 852 men, aged 40 to 59, resident in Zutphen and free from coronary heart disease (as of 1960), followed up over the next 20-year period.

   b. The efficiency increases.

   c. It would give an underestimation of the relative risk (RR→0). This is avoided if the comparison is based on incidence rate.

   d. Of the 20, a number were excluded because they had coronary heart disease at the start of the follow-up period (1960). Others were lost because complete information about exposure and potential confounders was not obtained in the examination in 1960.

   e. Regarding dietary habits, it should be borne in mind that a low fish consumption may mean, for example, a high meat consumption. (The alternative to eating a lot of fish may be to eat more of something else.) The covariance between different dietary habits means that particular attention must be paid to the possibility of confounding from other dietary factors that may influence the risk of coronary heart disease. In the current investigation account was taken of, for example, energy intake, monounsaturated and polyunsaturated fat intake, dietary cholesterol, animal protein, polysaccharides, and alcohol. Other potential confounders include age, smoking, systolic blood pressure, serum cholesterol, obesity, physical activity, and occupation. It was seen, however, that only a few of these factors were covariant with fish consumption and also influenced the risk of death from coronary heart disease. In the investigation in question, controlling for confounding from these factors in the data analysis did not result in any appreciable change in the observed association.

f. Nondifferential misclassification of exposed as unexposed and vice versa would lead to an underestimation of the strength of the association. Misclassification of low exposed as high exposed, or vice versa, would result in the strength of the association being underestimated among the high exposed, or overestimated among the low exposed, respectively.

   The effect, if any, of a nondifferential misclassification with respect to disease (cause of death) would be an underestimation of the strength of the association. This would not apply if the misclassification were differential, i.e., if the diagnosis of coronary heart disease in the event of death differs form individuals with a high or low fish consumption, respectively (which seems here to be unlikely). However, an investigation where, for example, individuals with a high fish consumption live in a rural area and individuals with a low fish consumption in an urban area, and the post mortem frequency is higher in the urban area, there is the possibility of an underdiagnosis of coronary heart disease in the rural area (i.e., among individuals with a high fish consumption).

g. In a subdivision into five exposure levels, the precision will be relatively low (the confidence intervals wide). If the data were collapsed into a smaller number of exposure levels, the precision at each level would increase.

(Kromhout D et al: The inverse relation between fish consumption and 20-year mortality from coronary heart disease. *N Engl J Med* 1985;312:1205-9.)

9. a. Because they already had the studied disease at the start of the follow-up period, or because of potential confounders such as dysplasia (i.e., restriction in the choice of the study base).

   b. Nonparticipation in the follow-up with respect to disease occurrence.

   c. The follow-up period was 6 years (starting in 1979). Of the 846 women who returned for a repeat smear after 1979, a large proportion could not be followed up until the end of the period on account of their not turning up for further smears ($6 \times 846 = 5,076$ person-years, whereas the follow-up comprised 3,448 person-years).

   d. The number of person-years lost to follow-up among the exposed was $(6 \times 261) + (5,076 - 3,448) = 3,194$ person-years. If the incidence was lower among the women who were lost to repeat smears, this would result in an overestimation of RR.

   e. Age-specific incidence rates from an adjacent state were used. The comparability depends on this state being similar to Victoria in terms of age-specific incidence (no potential confounders were taken into account except age). Occurrence of exposure (papilloma virus infection) in the adjacent state may have resulted in a certain underestimation of the strength of the association. A similar effect may be expected due to the occurrence of, for example, dysplasia in the adjacent state (compare *a*).

f. The follow-up of the exposed (3,448 person-years) was carried out with relatively frequent cervical smears. If the follow-up with respect to disease incidence was less intense in the adjacent state, this may have resulted in an overestimation of RR.

g. Nondifferential misclassification would given an underestimation of the strength of the association (RR→1). It was seen, however, that the cytological findings considered typical of infection with human papilloma virus were sometimes difficult to distinguish from mild dysplasia. If this resulted in women with mild dysplasia being included among the exposed, this would lead to an overestimation of RR if the incidence among women with mild dysplasia was higher than among women with human papilloma virus infection. A supplementary investigation in Victoria established, among other things, that of 86 women with mild dysplasia, 23 developed carcinoma *in situ* within 4 years. A relatively small proportion (less than 10%) with mild dysplasia among the exposed might therefore explain the observed association.

(Mitchell H et al: Prospective evaluation of risk of cervical cancer after cytological evidence of human papilloma virus infection. *Lancet* 1986;1:573-5.)

10. a. A total of 782 men who had initially reported physician-diagnosed coronary heart disease were excluded from the study (restriction). They had a higher mortality rate but did not differ much from other men in terms of physical activity. A separate analysis showed that the results of the investigation would not have been altered appreciably if they had not been excluded. A smaller group of men with cancer, stroke, or other ailments were not excluded.

b. In an investigation of total mortality, a preventive effect on mortality from some diseases could be balanced by an opposite effect, or diluted by the absence of effect, on mortality from other diseases. The impact on the association between physical activity and total mortality depends on the direction and strength of the association (if any) between physical activity and mortality from specific diseases, and on the proportion of all deaths contributed by the specific diseases. In the present study, the underlying causes of death were cardiovascular disease in 45%, cancer in 32%, other natural causes in 13%, and trauma in 10% of the cases. A decline in death rates with increasing physical activity was seen for each cause but was strongest in relation to cardiovascular and respiratory diseases.

c. It would give an underestimation of the strength of the association (RR→1). However, the effect will be limited unless there are great variations in physical activity over a period of time. In the investigation, the follow-up period was divided into three parts. For every such period a similar association between physical activity and mortality was observed. (This was considered, moreover, to argue against the possibility of confounding from diseases present at the start of the follow-up period.)

d. Some factor (which was not investigated) that is greatly covariant with physical activity and influences the risk of dying from several of the most common causes of death, particularly cardiovascular and respiratory diseases.

(Paffenbarger RS et al: Physical activity, all-cause mortality, and longevity of college alumni. *N Engl J Med,* 1986;314:605–13.)

11. a. No difference in terms of validity (provided that the interview data were handled blind). The case-control design is likely to be more efficient. The extent to which the efficiency increases depends on the incidence of the disease and on the cost per individual for the encoding and processing of primary data from the interviews.

   b. Alternative II may give a greater nondifferential misclassification with respect to dietary habits 5 years prior to the follow-up period. The extent of the misclassification depends on, among other things, the change in dietary habits during the 5-year period and how this influences misclassification with the use of retrospective dietary information in accordance with alternative II. This may give some underestimation of the strength of the association, i.e., influence the relative risk toward RR=1 (see Tables section). Alternative II is likely to be more efficient (lower-cost because of every individual being interviewed only once).

   c. With alternative III the disease might influence the quality of the exposure information. The likelihood of this depends on, for example, the studied association being "known" by the cases and whether the disease has altered the dietary habits (and consequently the quality of the information on past dietary habits) when the cases are interviewed. The effect may be an over- or underestimation of the relative risk. Alternative III is likely to be considerably more efficient (substantially fewer individuals are interviewed).

   d. Alternative IV may lead to a higher participation rate among the controls (and perhaps also greater similarity between cases and controls in terms of the quality of the exposure information). This must be weighed against the fact that the choice of controls may introduce a systematic error into the investigation (see Chapter 9).

12. In a type B case-control study, the disease (colon cancer) could affect the blood lipids and, consequently, the information on exposure during an etiologically relevant period. (This may occur before the disease is diagnosed, and thus may also be a problem during the first part of the follow-up period in Example 7.1).

13. a. Individuals aged 20 to 79 in a defined catchment area during a 4-year period.

    b. An open population.

    c. Skin pigmentation, sun habits, and other factors that may influence the risk of melanoma and that are conceivably covariant with the exposure (dysplastic nevi).

    d. If the presence of several dysplastic nevi increases the probability of being examined with respect to melanoma (e.g., through removal and microscopic examination of "melanoma-suspect" nevi), this may result in a larger proportion of early, slowly growing melanomas being diagnosed. This would result in an overestimation of the relative risk.

    e. If the person conducting the macro- and microscopic examinations to identify dysplastic nevi knows which individuals are cases and controls, respectively, this may influence the identification of dysplastic nevi. If the probability of identifying dysplastic nevi is greater for cases than for controls, this results in an overestimation of the relative risk. (To avoid this, the examination with respect to dysplastic nevi was conducted blind.)

f. The advantage would be that the disease (malignant melanoma) cannot influence the classification with respect to exposure (dysplastic nevi). The disadvantage would be that the efficiency of the investigation would decrease considerably as a result of the primary data having to be collected from a very large number of individuals.

g. A potential advantage is that the participation rate among the controls might be higher. The disadvantage is the difficulty in finding a control group that reflects the exposure frequency in the study base.

14. The studied psychological factors should not influence the risk of developing the disease(s) of the controls or the probability of those who fall ill being hospitalized (see Chapter 9). The second condition in particular may give rise to problems, unless controls with diseases that always lead to hospitalization are chosen. Naturally, the controls should also be chosen in such a way that the individuals can be examined with respect to exposure conditions (interviews, tests, etc.).

15. a. If the study base is defined as "all subjects aged 65 to 79 resident in the catchment area in question during a 2-year period," one may wonder whether the identified cases represent all incident cases of cataract in the study base. Mild cataract is common among older people and does not always lead to visits to an eye clinic. The probability of examination and diagnosis at the eye clinic may be influenced by exposure conditions. The study base is therefore better defined as "the subjects aged 65 to 79 resident in the catchment area in question, who would have received the diagnosis of cataract at the eye clinic in question if they had developed the disease during a 2-year period."

b. The study base in question is not available for random sampling. It is doubtful that, for example, neighbors of the cases would be a more suitable control group than a random sample from the population in the catchment area during the follow-up period. (The problem is that the identified cases may not reflect the exposure frequency among all cases.) One possibility is to try to find hospital controls that reflect the exposure frequency in the study base in question. This presupposes that the exposure does not influence the risk of developing the disease(s) of the controls and also that the exposure influences the probability of hospitalization equally for cases and controls (see Chapter 9). The latter condition may be difficult to fulfill.

c. One possibility is to choose the cases (and the study base) in another way, for example, pronounced cataract (in accordance with certain criteria) in the 40–59-year age group (who are more frequently called for examination by a specialist), and to use information from, among others, eye specialists in the primary health care service and in private practice to identify all cases that occur in the age group in the catchment area during the follow-up period. The controls can then be selected as a random sample of the study base. The fact that the investigation is limited to younger individuals does not necessarily mean that the efficiency decreases (see Chapter 4). Another possibility is to conduct the investigation as a type A case-control study, or possibly a cohort study, but this would reduce considerably the efficiency of the investigation.

16. a. A closed population.

b. Yes. The subjects (maternity records) could be identified via the register.

c. Both precision and cost increase with the number of controls selected (see Chapter 6). Taking this into account, four times as many controls as cases were selected in the study.

d. The efficiency may be somewhat improved. (Sex was a relatively strong risk indicator for the disease.) The controls were matched to the cases on the basis of, among other things, sex.

e. Maternity records were a useful source of information since they were available for both the cases and the controls. This information was, in addition, collected at the start of the follow-up period. (On the other hand, the case records would be an unsuitable source of information since there is no corresponding source of information for the controls. Use of such information would result in differential exposure misclassification.) Information about, for example, the length of gestation was found in all the maternity records. The infant's sex, length of gestation, birth order, and other drugs taken by mother or infant were seen not to influence the observed association between Bendectin and pyloric stenosis. Information about smoking habits was lacking for about 50%, and it was therefore considered impossible to take smoking into account in the analysis. A subdivision of exposure based on different periods of time during pregnancy suggested that the effect was most appreciable following exposure during weeks 8 to 10.

f. A type A case-control study.

(Aselton P et al: Pyloric stenosis and maternal Bendectin exposure. *Am J Epidemiol* 1984;120:251-6.)

17. a. The study base comprises the women who had never smoked in the 1961 and 1963 surveys followed up

during the period 1961–80 and 1963–80, respectively. The study population is closed. The investigation is a type B case-control study since the exposure information (passive smoking) was collected after the cases had been identified.

b. The considerably greater effect of smoking might conceal the effect of passive smoking among women who themselves were or had been smokers. In the investigation information about smoking habits in the 1961 and 1963 surveys was supplemented with questions about smoking in the 1984 survey. Only 1.8% were identified as smokers in the 1984 survey (these were excluded). This suggests that with the 1961 and 1963 surveys practically all women who had smoked were excluded.

c. Exposure of the lower respiratory tract (lungs) to tobacco smoke from other smokers (theoretically defined) and marriage to a smoker (empirically measured). Some of the women who had not been married to smokers may have been exposed to passive smoking (e.g., at their places of work), which would result in an underestimation of the strength of the association ($RR \rightarrow 1$). If the cases (or their next of kin) were more inclined to report smoking by their husbands than the controls (the association between smoking and lung cancer is generally known), this would produce an overestimation of the relative risk. The argument against this, however, is the fact that no excess risk was found for other primary lung cancers than for squamous and small-cell carcinoma.

d. $RR=2.0$ and $RR=1.4$, respectively (instead of $RR=3.5$). For 15 added cases (total number of controls=k):

	Exposed	Unexposed
Cases	x	$15-x$
Controls	$0.4 \times k$	$0.6 \times k$

$RR = 1$, i.e.,

$$\frac{x \times 0.6 \times k}{(15-x) \times 0.4 \times k} = 1; \qquad x = 6$$

With the 15 added cases (6 exposed, 9 unexposed):

	Exposed	Unexposed
Cases	$14+6$	$6+9$
Controls	$0.4 \times k$	$0.6 \times k$

$$RR = \frac{(14+6) \times 0.6 \times k}{(6+9) \times 0.4 \times k} = 2.0$$

e. In the 1984 survey, information about occupation and residence (degree of urbanization and risk of radon exposure in the home) was collected. However, these factors were seen not to be confounders in the data analysis. The exposed group included only women who had been married, whereas the unexposed group also included women who had not been married. This could explain the observed association only if the risk of certain types of lung cancer is considerably lower among unmarried women than among women married to nonsmokers, which is unlikely.

(Pershagen G et al: Passive smoking and lung cancer in Swedish women. Am J Epidemiol 1987;125:17-24.)

18. a. A type C case-control study, using information from the surgical controls and from the neighborhood controls (unless all cases occurring in a study population that could be identified from the voting lists were identified in the 19 surgical wards, and the neighbor-

hood controls were selected as a random sample of this study population during the follow-up period 1975–78). If the cases were identified in such a way that the corresponding study base was not available for random sampling, the selection of controls is a problem in that it may introduce a systematic error (Chapter 9).

b. Because BMI may be related to such diseases. If so, surgical controls with these diseases would not reflect the exposure (BMI) distribution in the study base, i.e., the person-time that generated the cases.

c. Although some surgical patients were excluded, there could still be differences in BMI between surgical controls and the study base. Neighborhood controls could be better in this respect, but the selection of controls could always introduce a systematic error unless they are a random sample of the study base. The surgical controls had a higher response rate than the neighborhood controls. In addition, there may be differences with respect to exposure misclassification.

d. BMI was calculated on the basis of "recent" weight. The current disease could have reduced BMI among cases and some of the surgical controls. Thus, they were asked about their weight before the illness began. This could have introduced differences in the quality of information on BMI prior to the development of breast cancer in the cases and at a corresponding point in time for the neighborhood controls, and perhaps also for the surgical controls.

e. The following potential confounders were taken into account in the data analysis: ages at menarche, first birth, and menopause; number of births; years of education; previous benign breast disease; and family history of breast cancer.

(Lubin F et al: Overweight and changes in weight throughout adult life in breast cancer etiology: a case-control study. *Am J Epidemiol* 1985;122:579-88.)

19. a. A type C case-control study, since the controls were chosen among dead individuals and not at random from the study base (the living).

   b. Dead controls were chosen to achieve similarity to the cases regarding the premises for the collection of exposure information. The choice of dead controls introduces a systematic error into the investigation if the risk of (being identified as) dying from a cause related to arteriosclerotic heart disease is influenced by the studied exposure (intake of vitamin A).

   c. RR=1.6 (rather than RR=1.7). Examined (total number of controls=k):

	Exposed	Unexposed
Cases	a	b
Controls	$0.5 \times k$	$0.5 \times k$

   $$RR = 1.7; \quad \frac{a \times 0.5 \times k}{b \times 0.5 \times k} = 1.7; \quad a = 1.7 \times b$$

   Nonresponders (25%, i.e., one-third as many as the 75% examined) with exposure frequency one-half of that for the examined, for both cases and controls:

	Exposed	Unexposed
Cases	$(1/3)(1/2)1.7b$	$(1/3)[b+(1/2) 1.7b]$
Controls	$(1/3)(1/2)0.5k$	$(1/3)[0.5k+(1/2)0.5k]$

Total (examined+nonresponders):

	Exposed	Unexposed
Cases	1.7b+(1/3) (1/2)1.7b	b+(1/3)[b+ (1/2)1.7b]
Controls	0.5k+(1/3) (1/2)0.5k)	0.5k+(1/3) [0.5k+(1/2) 0.5k]

which gives RR=1.6.

d. To achieve comparability between cases and controls in terms of the quality of the exposure information (and, consequently, a misclassification that is independent of the disease), identical routines were implemented in the collection of data, and the interviewer did not know who were next of kin of the cases and the controls, respectively. To avoid differential misclassification, it may also be advisable to collect exposure information for a similar proportion of the cases as of the controls each month, since there may be considerable seasonal variations in the intake of vitamin A, and this may influence the exposure information. The intake of vitamin A may display great variation from day to day, which may lead to considerable nondifferential misclassification (RR→1) if the exposure information refers to a short time. If sufficient account has not been taken of the induction period, this, too, may produce an underestimation of the strength of the association (RR→1).

e. Dietary factors (vitamin C, fibers?) that are covariant with vitamin A in the diet and may conceivably influence the risk of stomach cancer. In the investigation account was taken of, for example, tobacco, alcohol, socioeconomic status, occupation, and county of residence.

(Stehr PA et al: Dietary vitamin A deficiency and stomach cancer. *Am J Epidemiol* 1985;121:65-70.)

20. a. A type C case-control study. The study base was "those men in the 20–54 age group, without earlier cardiac diseases or angina pectoris, who would have been treated for myocardial infarction at one of the 78 hospitals if they had developed a myocardial infarction during the period 1980–83."

    b. To avoid confounding from earlier cardiac disease and angina pectoris, which may influence both the risk of myocardial infarction and the inclination to stop smoking.

    c. Yes, if the smoking habits influence the probability of those who have developed the diseases in the controls being treated at the hospitals in question. Among the controls there were, for example, men who had been treated for gastrointestinal disorders (20%) and other conditions (23%), some of which do not always lead to hospitalization. The proportion of smokers among the controls was also reported to be somewhat higher than in the population at large. This may have led to a certain underestimation of the relative risk for smokers. If the probability of hospitalization (among men who developed the diseases in the controls) was lower for men who had never smoked and/or higher for men who had stopped smoking, this might produce an underestimation of the relative risk for men who have stopped smoking.

    d. Account should be taken of the fact that smoking habits may have differed for men who had stopped or had not stopped smoking, respectively. In the investigation a subdivision was therefore made based on the intensity of the smoking (number of cigarettes/day) and duration (number of years). The relative risk for smokers increased with the number of cigarettes per day (RR=4.1 for at least 25 cigarettes/day). Regardless of the intensity and duration of smoking, however, excess risks were found for men who had smoked during the last 12 months and for men who had quit smoking 12 to 23 months previously, but not for men who had quit smoking at least 2 years previously.

The association between smoking and myocardial infarction is generally known. If the cases who were smokers were less inclined because of this to state that they had stopped smoking, compared with the corresponding controls, this would result in an underestimation of the relative risk for men who have stopped smoking. A nondifferential misclassification with respect to exposure might produce a certain underestimation of the strength of the association (RR→1).

e. In the investigation, account was taken of, for example, overweight (body mass index=weight (kg)/ height $(m)^2 > 26$), history of elevated serum cholesterol level, history of myocardial infarction or stroke in parent or sibling before the age of 60, physical activity, so-called type A personality, education (number of years), number of medical visits in the previous year, and geographic location of the hospital. These factors were seen, however, to have little influence on the observed association. Moreover, the effect of quitting smoking was observed for individuals with or without excess weight, elevated serum cholesterol, etc.

(Rosenberg L et al: The risk of myocardial infarction after quitting smoking in men under 55 years of age. *N Engl J Med* 1985;313:1511-4.)

References

Listed here are examples of the available literature on study design, validity, and efficiency in epidemiology. (The numbers refer to the references in the reference section.)

Confounding

4, 18, 21, 26, 72, 184, 215, 217, 237, 239, 241, 243, 244, 259, 283, 354, 400, 401, 407, 410, 412, 414, 418, 426, 471, 493, 494, 526, 536, 545, 565, 569, 597, 660, 670, 676, 692

Classification, Misclassification

Exposure:

6, 20, 23, 34, 36, 37, 44, 52, 62, 69, 73, 75, 76, 85, 86, 105, 107, 109, 110, 118, 123, 128, 146, 176, 182, 200, 205, 223, 225, 233, 235, 243, 251, 254, 257, 258, 261, 262, 264, 268, 270, 273, 276, 280, 299, 304, 306, 317, 327, 328, 334, 340, 343, 349, 351, 353, 355, 372, 375, 380, 384, 395, 399, 430, 467, 476, 477, 479, 480, 481, 485, 486, 501, 505, 506, 513, 514, 517, 522, 523, 545, 554, 574, 583, 584, 589, 601, 615, 617, 639, 644, 646, 667, 670, 671, 678, 689, 701

Diet factors

33, 57, 58, 59, 60, 88, 89, 90, 102, 111, 129, 131, 136, 142, 177, 192, 193, 274, 285, 289, 290, 292, 300, 302, 303, 350, 352, 367, 383,

386, 396, 433, 434, 448, 478, 487, 488, 515, 516, 543, 551, 581, 600, 613, 635, 647, 648, 655, 656, 657, 658, 696, 697, 698, 699, 703, 704

Disease

3, 13, 28, 34, 38, 39, 41, 43, 48, 53, 55, 71, 84, 93, 97, 98, 99, 106, 108, 109, 115, 116, 119, 121, 143, 144, 156 (bibliography), 175, 181, 183, 190, 198, 204, 235, 242, 243, 248, 252, 255, 260, 269, 275, 278, 279, 293, 313, 321, 323, 331, 332, 333, 340, 342, 356, 365, 369, 374, 381, 382, 388, 389, 390, 392, 405, 431, 438, 439, 440, 447, 450, 457, 468, 474, 498, 500, 507, 512, 520, 542, 545, 550, 552, 562, 576, 591, 592, 604, 607, 608, 609, 611, 612, 618, 620, 622, 628, 642, 645, 646, 672, 674, 680, 688, 691, 693

Confounders

199, 223, 243, 340, 558, 664

Nonresponse

12, 42, 47, 64, 103, 114, 122, 124, 125, 126, 222, 256, 379, 441, 517, 578, 585, 606, 613, 675, 684

Precision, Efficiency

2, 56, 68, 80, 94, 100, 127, 135, 232, 348, 406, 418, 437, 443, 459, 463, 466, 483, 489, 495, 496, 536, 553, 564, 566, 568, 589, 596, 634, 636, 637, 638

Matching in Case-Control Studies

22, 240, 284, 310, 408, 409, 418, 536, 553, 566, 634, 638

Choice of Controls

16, 24, 25, 49, 104, 112, 155, 165, 169, 174, 194, 210, 227, 246, 253, 256, 278, 286, 293, 296, 326, 366, 371, 373, 397, 398, 403, 416,

418, 419, 420, 428, 454, 458, 470, 490, 521, 536, 559, 566, 567, 573, 587, 588, 591, 594, 610, 661, 669, 687, 690

Experimental Studies

12, 17, 79, 81, 82, 87, 91, 113, 117, 120, 133, 137, 150, 151, 173, 191, 195, 202, 218, 249, 288, 385, 417, 482, 491, 492, 529, 535, 546, 548, 561, 586, 598, 629, 649, 651, 705, 706

Causality

3, 45, 83, 147, 148, 152, 160, 186, 216, 231, 267, 277, 294, 295, 309, 319, 338, 361, 432, 510, 511, 522, 527, 536, 538, 556, 570, 575, 603, 624, 631, 682, 685

Effect Modification

21, 61, 237, 271, 329, 330, 341, 412, 418, 471, 525, 528, 530, 531, 536, 539, 555, 590, 597, 670, 673, 683

Ethics, Philosophy

9, 10, 14, 15, 29, 31, 35, 46, 67, 77, 78, 130, 139, 167, 168, 196, 197, 208, 211, 212, 214, 219, 265, 291, 301, 307, 339, 376, 377, 422, 472, 508, 534, 540, 561, 593, 602, 625, 626, 633, 652, 653, 679

REFERENCE LIST

1. Abramson JH. Classification of epidemiologic research. *J Clin Epidemiol* 1989;42:819–20.
2. Adams MJ Jr, Khoury MJ, James LM. The use of attributable fraction in the design and interpretation of epidemiologic studies. *J Clin Epidemiol* 1989;42:659–62.
3. Ahlbom A, Norell SE. Introduction to modern epidemiology (second edition). Epidemiology Resources Inc., Chestnut Hill, 1990.
4. Albanes D. Potential for confounding of physical activity risk assessment by body weight and fatness. *Am J Epidemiol* 1987;125:745–6.

5. Ales KL, Charlson ME. In search of the true inception cohort. *J Chron Dis* 1987;40:881–5.
6. Alexander GR, Petersen DJ, Powell-Griner E, Tompkins ME. A comparison of gestational age reporting methods based on physician estimate and date of last normal menses from fetal death reports. *Am J Pub Health* 1989;79:600–2.
7. Alwall N. Population studies on non-obstructive urinary tract infection in non-pregnant women: importance of method and material. *Acta Med Scand* 1978;203:95–105.
8. Anderson DW, Mantel N. On epidemiologic surveys. *Am J Epidemiol* 1983;118:613–9.
9. Angell M. Negative studies. *N Engl J Med* 1989;321:464–6.
10. Angell M, Relman AS. Redundant publication. *N Engl J Med* 1989; 320:1212–4.
11. Anonymous. Improving data bases for international studies. *Int J Epidemiol* 1984;13:267–8.
12. Anonymous. Drop-outs from clinical trials. *Lancet* 1987a;2:892–3.
13. Anonymous. Cancer cytogenetics in clinical diagnosis. *Lancet* 1987b; 2:1186.
14. Anonymous. Peers reviewed. *Lancet* 1989a;1:1115–6.
15. Anonymous. The *Journal's* peer-review process. *N Engl J Med* 1989b; 321:837–9.
16. Armenian HK, Lakkis NG, Sibai AM, Halabi SS. Hospital visitors as controls. *Am J Epidemiol* 1988;127:404–6.
17. Armitage P. Inference and decision in clinical trials. *J Clin Epidemiol* 1989;42:293–9.
18. Austin H. The identification of confounders in case-control studies. *J Chron Dis* 1983;36:309–10.
19. Axelson O. The case-referent (case-control) study in occupational health epidemiology. *Scand J Work Environ Health* 1979;5:91–9.
20. Axelson O. A note on observational bias in case-referent studies in occupational health epidemiology. *Scand J Work Environ Health* 1980;6:80–2.
21. Axelson O. Elucidation of some epidemiologic principles. *Scand J Work Environ Health* 1983;9:231–40.
22. Axelson O. The case-referent study—some comments on its structure, merits and limitations. *Scand J Work Environ Health* 1985a;11: 207–13.
23. Axelson O. Dealing with the exposure variable in occupational and environmental epidemiology. *Scand J Soc Med* 1985b;13:147–52.
24. Axelson O. The "case-control" study: valid selection of subjects. *J Chron Dis* 1985c;38:553–5.
25. Axelson O, Flodin U, Hardell L. A comment on the reference series with regard to multiple exposure evaluations in a case-referent study. *Scand J Work Environ Health* 1982;8(suppl 1):15–9.
26. Axelson O, Johansson B, Axelson T. On the problem of controlling confounding in case-referent studies. *Ann Acad Med* (Singapore) 1984;13(suppl):308–11.
27. Axelsson G, Rylander R. Exposure to anaesthetic gases and sponta-

neous abortion: Response bias in a postal questionnaire study. *Int J Epidemiol* 1982;11:250–6.

28. Axelsson G, Rylander R. Validation of questionnaire reported miscarriage, malformation and birth weight. *Int J Epidemiol* 1984;13:94–8.
29. Bailar JC III. Research quality, methodologic rigor, citation counts, and impact. *Am J Pub Health* 1982;72:1103–4.
30. Bailar JC III. When research results are in conflict. *N Engl J Med* 1985;313:1080–1.
31. Bailar JC III, Louis TA, Lavori PW, Polansky M. A classification for biomedical research reports. *N Engl J Med* 1984;311:1482–7.
32. Bain C, Colditz GA, Willett WC et al. Self-reports of mole counts and cutaneous malignant melanoma in women: methodological issues and risk of disease. *Am J Epidemiol* 1988;127:703–12.
33. Bakkum A, Bloemberg B, van Staveren WA et al. The relative validity of a retrospective estimate of food consumption based on a current dietary history and a food frequency list. *Nutr Cancer* 1988;11:41–53.
34. Barron BA. The effects of misclassification on the estimation of relative risk. *Biometrics* 1977;33:414–8.
35. Baum M. Do we need informed consent? *Lancet* 1986;2:911–2.
36. Bauman KE, Koch GG, Bryan ES et al. On the measurement of tobacco use by adolescents. *Am J Epidemiol* 1989;130:327–37.
37. Baumgarten M, Siemiatycki J, Gibbs GW. Validity of work histories obtained by interview for epidemiologic purposes. *Am J Epidemiol* 1983;118:583–91.
38. Beaglehole R, Stewart AW, Butler M. Comparability of old and new World Health Organization criteria for definite myocardial infarction. *Int J Epidemiol* 1987;16:373–6.
39. Becklake MR, Freeman S, Goldsmith C et al. Respiratory questionnaires in occupational studies: their use in multilingual workforces on the Witwatersrand. *Int J Epidemiol* 1987;16:606–11.
40. Beebe GW. Long-term follow-up is a problem. *Am J Pub Health* 1983;73:245–6.
41. Begg CB, Greenes RA, Iglewicz B. The influence of uninterpretability on the assessment of diagnostic tests. *J Chron Dis* 1986;39:575–84.
42. Benfante R, Reed D, MacLean C, Kagan A. Response bias in the Honolulu heart program. *Am J Epidemiol* 1989;130:1088–1100.
43. Benn RT, Leck I, Nwene UP. Estimation of completeness of cancer registration. *Int J Epidemiol* 1982;11:362–7.
44. Beresford SAA, Coker AL. Pictorially assisted recall of past hormone use in case-control studies. *Am J Epidemiol* 1989;130:202–5.
45. Berg AT, Herman AA. Causality inference in observational vs experimental studies: an empirical comparison. *Am J Epidemiol* 1989;130:206.
46. Berger PM, Stallones RA. Legal liability and epidemiologic research. *Am J Epidemiol* 1977;106:177–83.
47. Bergstrand R, Vedin A, Wilhelmsson C, Wilhelmsen L. Bias due to non-participation and heterogenous sub-groups in population surveys. *J Chron Dis* 1983;36:725–8.

48. Berkman PL. Measurement of mental health in a general population survey. *Am J Epidemiol* 1971;94:105–11.
49. Berkson J. Limitations of the application of fourfold table analysis to hospital data. *Biometrics* 1946;2:47–53.
50. Bertazzi P-A. Industrial disasters and epidemiology. A review of recent experiences. *Scand J Work Environ Health* 1989;15: 85–100.
51. Biersteker K, Schouten EG, Kok FJ. Weak associations in epidemiology—introduction. *Int J Epidemiol* 1988;17:949.
52. Birkett NJ. Computer-aided personal interviewing. A new technique for data collection in epidemiologic surveys. *Am J Epidemiol* 1988a; 127:684–90.
53. Birkett NJ. Evaluation of diagnostic tests with multiple diagnostic categories. *J Clin Epidemiol* 1988b;41:491–4.
54. Birnbaum A. On the foundations of statistical inference. *J Am Stat Assoc* 1962;57:269–326.
55. Bland JM, Altman DG. Statistical methods for assessing agreement between two methods of clinical measurement. *Lancet* 1986;1: 307–10.
56. Blitzer PH, Hsieh C-C, Miettinen OS. Power calculation in matched case-referent studies. Application and accuracy of the asymptotic power function. *Am J Epidemiol* 1986;124:836–42.
57. Block G. A review of validations of dietary assessment methods. *Am J Epidemiol* 1982;115:492–505.
58. Block G, Hartman AM, Dresser CM et al. A data-based approach to diet questionnaire design and testing. *Am J Epidemiol* 1986;124: 453–69.
59. Bloemberg BPM, Kromhout D, Obermann-De Boer GL. The relative validity of retrospectively assessed energy intake data in cases with myocardial infarction and controls (the Zutphen study). *J Clin Epidemiol* 1989;42:1075–82.
60. Bloemberg BPM, Kromhout D, Obermann-De Boer GL, Van Kampen-Donker M. The reproducibility of dietary intake data assessed with the cross-check dietary history method. *Am J Epidemiol* 1989;130:1047–56.
61. Blot WJ, Day NE. Synergism and interaction: are they equivalent? *Am J Epidemiol* 1979;110:99–100.
62. Bond GG, Bodner KM, Sobel W et al. Validation of work histories obtained from interviews. *Am J Epidemiol* 1988;128:343–51.
63. Brady WF, Martinoff JT. Validity of health history data collected from dental patients and patient perception of health status. *J Am Dent Assoc* 1980;101:642–5.
64. Brambilla DJ, McKinlay SM. A comparison of responses to mailed questionnaires and telephone interviews in a mixed mode health survey. *Am J Epidemiol* 1987;126:962–71.
65. Breslow NE, Day NE. Statistical methods in cancer research. Vol 1. The analysis of case-control studies. International Agency for Research on Cancer, Lyon 1980.
66. Breslow NE, Day NE. Statistical methods in cancer research. Vol 2.

The design and analysis of cohort studies. International Agency for Research on Cancer, Lyon 1987.

67. Brigham KL. On being wrong in science. *N Engl J Med* 1985; 312: 794–5.
68. Brittain E, Schlesselman JJ, Stadel BV. Cost of case-control studies. *Am J Epidemiol* 1981;114:234–43.
69. Britten N. Validity of claims to lifelong non-smoking at age 36 in a longitudinal study. *Int J Epidemiol* 1988;17:525–9.
70. Brody DS. An analysis of patient recall of their therapeutic regimens. *J Chron Dis* 1980;33:57–63.
71. Bross I. Misclassification in 2 × 2 tables. *Biometrics* 1954;10:478–86.
72. Bross ID, Bross NS. Do atomic veterans have excess cancer? New results correcting for the healthy soldier bias. *Am J Epidemiol* 1987; 126:1042–50.
73. Brownson RC, Davis JR, Chang JC et al. A study of the accuracy of cancer risk factor information reported to a central registry compared with that obtained by interview. *Am J Epidemiol* 1989;129:616–24.
74. Brunekreef B, Dijkstra L, Fischer P, Houthuijs D. Weak associations in environmental epidemiology. *Int J Epidemiol* 1988;17(suppl): 960–3.
75. Brunekreef B, Noy D, Clausing P. Variability of exposure measurements, in environmental epidemiology. *Am J Epidemiol* 1987;125: 892–8.
76. Bryant HE, Visser N, Love EJ. Records, recall loss, and recall bias in pregnancy: a comparison of interview and medical records data of pregnant and postnatal women. *Am J Pub Health* 1989;79:78–80.
77. Buck C. Popper's philosophy for epidemiologists. *Int J Epidemiol* 1975;4:159–68.
78. Buck C. Problems with the Popperian approach: a response to Pearce and Crawford-Brown. *J Clin Epidemiol* 1989;42:185–7.
79. Buck C, Donner A. The design of controlled experiments in the evaluation of non-therapeutic interventions. *J Chron Dis* 1982;35:531–8.
80. Bulpitt CJ. Confidence intervals. *Lancet* 1987;1:494–7.
81. Bulpitt CJ. Subgroup analysis. *Lancet* 1988a;2:31–4.
82. Bulpitt CJ. Meta-analysis. *Lancet* 1988b;2:93–4.
83. Burch PRJ. The surgeon general's "epidemiologic criteria for causality". A critique. *J Chron Dis* 1983;36:821–36.
84. Burke GL, Edlavitch SA, Crow RS. The effects of diagnostic criteria on trends in coronary heart disease morbidity: the Minnesota heart survey. *J Clin Epidemiol* 1989;42:17–24.
85. Burke GL, Webber LS, Shear CL et al. Sources of error in measurement of children's blood pressure in a large epidemiologic study: Bogalusa heart study. *J Chron Dis* 1987;40:83–9.
86. Burns TL, Moll PP, Rost CA, Lauer RM. Mothers remember birthweights of adolescent children: the Muscatine ponderosity family study. *Int J Epidemiol* 1987;16:550–5.
87. Byar DP, Simon RM, Friedewald WT, et al. Randomized clinical trials. Perspectives on some recent ideas. *N Engl J Med* 1976;295: 74–80.

88. Byers T, Marshall J, Anthony E. et al. The reliability of dietary history from the distant past. *Am J Epidemiol* 1987;125:999–1011.

89. Byers T, Marshall J, Fiedler R et al. Assessing nutrient intake with an abbreviated dietary interview. *Am J Epidemiol* 1985;122:41–50.

90. Byers TE, Rosenthal RI, Marshall JR et al. Dietary history from the distant past: a methodological study. *Nutr Cancer* 1983;5:69–77.

91. Campbell DT, Stanley JC. Experimental and quasi-experimental designs for research. Rand McNally College Publishing Company, Chicago 1966.

92. Caper P. The epidemiologic surveillance of medical care. *Am J Pub Health* 1987;77:669–70.

93. Carter JR. The problematic death certificate. *N Engl J Med* 1985; 313:1285–6.

94. Casagrande JT, Pike MC, Smith PG. An improved approximate formula for calculating sample sizes for comparing two binomial distributions. *Biometrics* 1978;34:483–6.

95. Catalano R, Serxner S. Time series designs of potential interest to epidemiologists. *Am J Epidemiol* 1987;126:724–31.

96. Chamberlain G, Johnstone FD. Reliability of the history. *Lancet* 1975;1:103.

97. Chambers LW, Spitzer WO, Hill GB, Helliwell BE. Under-reporting of cancer in medical surveys: a source of systematic error in cancer research. *Am J Epidemiol* 1976;104:141–5.

98. Cherian T, John TJ, Simoes E et al. Evaluation of simple clinical signs for the diagnosis of acute lower respiratory tract infection. *Lancet* 1988;2:125–32.

99. Chinn S, Burney PGJ. On measuring repeatability of data from self-administered questionnaires. *Int J Epidemiol* 1987;16:121–7.

100. Choi BCK, Howe GR. Methodological issues in case-control studies: II. Test statistics as measures of efficiency. *Int J Epidemiol* 1984; 13:229–34.

101. Choi IC, Comstock GW. Interviewer effect on responses to a questionnaire relating to mood. *Am J Epidemiol* 1975;101:84–92.

102. Chu Sy, Kolonel LN, Hankin JH, Lee J. A comparison of frequency and quantitative dietary methods for epidemiologic studies of diet and disease. *Am J Epidemiol* 1984;119:323–34.

103. Clark VA, Aneshensel CS, Frerichs RR, Morgan TM. Analysis of non-response in a prospective study of depression in Los Angeles County. *Int J Epidemiol* 1983;12:193–8.

104. Clarke M, Clayton D. The design and interpretation of case-control studies of perinatal mortality. *Am J Epidemiol* 1981;113:636–45.

105. Coates RA, Calzavara LM, Soskolne CL et al. Validity of sexual histories in a prospective study of male sexual contacts of men with AIDS or an AIDS-related condition. *Am J Epidemiol* 1988;128:719–28.

106. Cochrane AL. The history of the measurement of ill health. *Int J Epidemiol* 1972;1:89–92.

107. Coghlin J, Hammond SK, Gann PH. Development of epidemiologic tools for measuring environmental tobacco smoke exposure. *Am J Epidemiol* 1989;130:696–704.

108. Cohen BB, Pokras R, Meads MS, Krushat WM. How will diagnosis-related groups affect epidemiologic research? *Am J Epidemiol* 1987; 126:1–9.
109. Colditz GA, Martin P, Stampfer MJ et al. Validation of questionnaire information on risk factors and disease outcomes in a prospective cohort study of women. *Am J Epidemiol* 1986;123:894–900.
110. Colditz GA, Stampfer MJ, Willett WC et al. Reproducibility and validity of self-reported menopausal status in a prospective cohort study. *Am J Epidemiol* 1987;126:319–25.
111. Colditz GA, Willett WC, Stampfer MJ et al. The influence of age, relative weight, smoking, and alcohol intake on the reproducibility of a dietary questionnaire. *Int J Epidemiol* 1987;16:392–8.
112. Cole P. The evolving case-control study. *J Chron Dis* 1979;32:15–27.
113. Comstock GW. Uncontrolled ruminations on modern controlled trials. *Am J Epidemiol* 1978;108:81–4.
114. Comstock GW, Helsing KJ. Characteristics of respondents and nonrespondents to a questionnaire for estimating community mood. *Am J Epidemiol* 1973;97:233–9.
115. Comstock GW, Markush RE. Further comments on problems in death certification. *Am J Epidemiol* 1986;124:180–1.
116. Connell FA, Koepsell TD. Measures of gain in certainty from a diagnostic test. *Am J Epidemiol* 1985;121:744–53.
117. Cook CCH, Scannell TD, Lipsedge MS. Another trial that failed. *Lancet* 1988;1:524–5.
118. Copeland KT, Checkoway H, McMichael AJ, Holbrook RH. Bias due to misclassification in the estimation of relative risk. *Am J Epidemiol* 1977;105:488–95.
119. Coren S, Hakstian AR. Validation of a self-report inventory for the measurement of visual acuity. *Int J Epidemiol* 1989;18:451–6.
120. Cornfield J. Randomization by group: a formal analysis. *Am J Epidemiol* 1978;108:100–2.
121. Corwin RG, Krober M, Roth HP. Patients' accuracy in reporting their past medical history, a study of 90 patients with peptic ulcer. *J Chron Dis* 1971;23:875–9.
122. Cottler LB, Zipp JF, Robins LN, Spitznagel EL. Difficult-to-recruit respondents and their effect on prevalence estimates in an epidemiologic survey. *Am J Epidemiol* 1987;125:329–39.
123. Coultas DB, Peake GT, Samet JM. Questionnaire assessment of lifetime and recent exposure to environmental tobacco smoke. *Am J Epidemiol* 1989;130:338–47.
124. Criqui MH. Response bias and risk ratios in epidemiologic studies. *Am J Epidemiol* 1979;109:394–9.
125. Criqui MH, Austin M, Barret-Connor E. The effect of non-response on risk ratios in a cardiovascular disease study. *J Chron Dis* 1979; 32:633–8.
126. Criqui MH, Barrett-Connor E, Austin M. Differences between respondents and non-respondents in a population-based cardiovascular disease study. *Am J Epidemiol* 1978;108:367–72.
127. Crombie IK. The limitations of case-control studies in the detection

of environmental carcinogens. *J Epidemiol Community Health* 1981; 35:281–7.

128. Cummings KM, Markello SJ, Mahoney MC, Marshall JR. Measurement of lifetime exposure to passive smoke. *Am J Epidemiol* 1989; 130:122–32.

129. Cummings SR, Block G, McHenry K, Baron RB. Evaluation of two food frequency methods of measuring dietary calcium intake. *Am J Epidemiol* 1987;126:796–802.

130. Davies AM. Comments on 'Popper's philosophy for epidemiologists' by Carol Buck. Comment one. *Int J Epidemiol* 1975;4:169–71.

131. Decker MD, Booth AL, Dewey MJ et al. Validity of food consumption histories in a foodborne outbreak investigation. *Am J Epidemiol* 1986;124:859–63.

132. de Waard F. Re: The relationship between Wolfe's classification of mammograms, accepted breast cancer risk factors, and the incidence of breast cancer. *Am J Epidemiol* 1987;125:171.

133. Diamond GA, Forrester JS. Clinical trials and statistical verdicts: probable grounds for appeal. *Ann Intern Med* 1983;98:385–94.

134. Doll R. Occupational cancer: a hazard for epidemiologists. *Int J Epidemiol* 1985;14:22–31.

135. Donner A. The number of families required for detecting the familial aggregation of a continuous attribute. *Am J Epidemiol* 1978;108: 425–8.

136. Dwyer JT, Gardner J, Halvorsen K et al. Memory of food intake in the distant past. *Am J Epidemiol* 1989;130:1033–46.

137. Ederer F. Practical problems in collaborative clinical trials. *Am J Epidemiol* 1975;102:111–8.

138. Edward AM, Schork MA, Harburg E et al. Sources of variability in quantitative levels of alcohol use in a total community: Sociodemographic and psychosocial correlates. *Int J Epidemiol* 1986;15: 82–90.

139. Eichorn P, Yankauer A. Do authors check their references? A survey of accuracy of references in three public health journals. *Am J Pub Health* 1987;77:1011–2.

140. Eklund G, Wiklund K. Quality control study of the personal identity in the cancer environment registry. National Central Bureau of Statistics, statistical review 1979. Third series, Vol. 17, 5, 373–6 and 407–8. Stockholm, Sweden.

141. Elandt-Johnson RC. Definition of rates: some remarks on their use and misuse. *Am J Epidemiol* 1975;102:267–71.

142. el Lozy M. Dietary variability and its impact on nutritional epidemiology. *J Chron Dis* 1983;36:237–49.

143. Engel LW, Strauchen JA, Chiazze L, Heid M. Accuracy of death certification in an autopsied population with specific attention to malignant neoplasms and vascular diseases. *Am J Epidemiol* 1980;111: 99–112.

144. Erdreich LS, Lee ET. Use of relative operating characteristic analysis in epidemiology. A method for dealing with subjective judgement. *Am J Epidemiol* 1981;114:649–62.

145. Esdaile JM, Horwitz RI. Observational studies of cause-effect rela-

tionships: an analysis of methodologic problems as illustrated by the conflicting data for the role of oral contraceptives in the etiology of rheumatoid arthritis. *J Chron Dis* 1986;39:841–52.

146. Eskenazi B, Pearson K. Validation of a self-administered questionnaire for assessing occupational and environmental exposures of pregnant women. *Am J Epidemiol* 1988;128:1117–29.

147. Evans AS. Causation and disease: the Henle-Koch postulates revisited. *Yale J Biol Med* 1976;49:175–95.

148. Evans AS. Causation and disease: a chronological journey. *Am J Epidemiol* 1978;108:249–58.

149. Evans AS. Subclinical epidemiology. *Am J Epidemiol* 1987;125:545–55.

150. Farquhar JW. The community-based model of life style intervention trials. *Am J Epidemiol* 1978;108:103–11.

151. Farr BM, Gwaltney JM Jr. The problems of taste in placebo matching: an evaluation of zinc gluconate for the common cold. *J Chron Dis* 1987;40:875–9.

152. Feinstein AR. Scientific standards vs statistical associations and biologic logic in the analysis of causation. *Clin Pharmacol Ther* 1979a;25:481–92.

153. Feinstein AR. Methodologic problems and standards in case-control research. *J Chron Dis* 1979b;32:35–41.

154. Feinstein AR. Experimental requirements and scientific principles in case-control studies. *J Chron Dis* 1985a;38:127–33.

155. Feinstein AR. The case-control study: valid selection of subjects. *J Chron Dis* 1985b;38:551–2.

156. Feinstein AR. A bibliography of publications on observer variability. *J Chron Dis* 1985c;38:619–32.

157. Feinstein AR. Directionality in epidemiologic research *J Clin Epidemiol* 1988a;41:705–7.

158. Feinstein AR. Classification of epidemiologic research. *J Clin Epidemiol* 1988b;41:805.

159. Feinstein AR. Models, methods, and goals. *J Clin Epidemiol* 1989a;42:301–8.

160. Feinstein AR. Epidemiologic analyses of causation: the unlearned scientific lessons of randomized trials. *J Clin Epidemiol* 1989b;42:481–9.

161. Feinstein AR. Unlearned lessons from clinical trials: a duality of outlooks. *J Clin Epidemiol* 1989c;42:497–8.

162. Feinstein AR. Directionality and scientific inference. *J Clin Epidemiol* 1989d;42:829–33.

163. Feinstein AR. Para-analysis, *faute de mieux,* and the perils of riding on a data barge. *J Clin Epidemiol* 1989e;42:929–35.

164. Feinstein AR, Horwitz RI. An algebraic analysis of biases due to exclusion, susceptibility, and protopathic prescription in case-control research. *J Chron Dis* 1981;34:393–403.

165. Feinstein AR, Horwitz RI. On choosing the control group in case-control studies. *J Chron Dis* 1983;36:311–3.

166. Feinstein AR, Horwitz RI, Spitzer WO, Battista RN. Coffee and

pancreatic cancer: the problems of etiologic science and epidemiologic case-control research. *JAMA* 1981;246:957–61.

167. Feinstein AR, Spitzer WO. The unknown reviewer: an expression of policy and gratitude. *J Chron Dis* 1987;40:101–4.

168. Feinstein AR, Spitzer WO. Who checks what in the divided responsibilities of editors and authors? *J Clin Epidemiol* 1988;41:945–8.

169. Feinstein AR, Walter SD, Horwitz RI. An analysis of Berkson's bias in case-control studies. *J Chron Dis* 1986;39:495–504.

170. Fett MJ. The development of matching criteria for epidemiological studies using record linkage techniques. *Int J Epidemiol* 1984;13:351–5.

171. Fett MJ. Measuring the accuracy of vital status data in cohort studies. *Am J Pub Health* 1985;75:1385–8.

172. Fisher L, Patil K. Matching and unrelatedness. *Am J Epidemiol* 1974;100:347–9.

173. Fisher RA. The Design of Experiments. Oliver and Boyd, Edinburgh 1925.

174. Flanders WD, Austin H. Possibility of selection bias in matched case-control studies using friend controls. *Am J Epidemiol* 1986;124:150–3.

175. Flanders WD, Boyle CA, Boring JR. Bias associated with differential hospitalization rates in incident case-control studies. *J Clin Epidemiol* 1989;42:395–401.

176. Flegal KM, Brownie C, Haas JD. The effects of exposure misclassification on estimates of relative risk. *Am J Epidemiol* 1986;123:736–51.

177. Flegal KM, Larkin FA, Metzner HL et al. Counting calories: partitioning energy intake estimates from a food frequency questionnaire. *Am J Epidemiol* 1988;128:749–60.

178. Fleiss JL. Significance tests have a role in epidemiologic research: reactions to AM Walker. *Am J Pub Health* 1986a;76:559–60.

179. Fleiss JL. Confidence intervals vs significance tests: quantitative interpretation. *Am J Pub Health* 1986b;76:587. Response from Drs. Foxman and Freirichs, and Editors' Note 587–8.

180. Florey C du V. Weak associations in epidemiological research: some examples and their interpretation. *Int J Epidemiol* 1988;17:950–4.

181. Folsom AR, Gomez-Marin O, Gillum RF et al. Out-of-hospital coronary death in an urban population—validation of death certificate diagnosis. *Am J Epidemiol* 1987;125:1012–8.

182. Foster TA, Berenson GS. Measurement error and reliability in four pediatric cross-sectional surveys of cardiovascular disease risk factor variables—the Bogalusa heart study. *J Chron Dis* 1987;40:13–21.

183. Fowkes FGR. The measurement of atherosclerotic peripheral arterial disease in epidemiological surveys. *Int J Epidemiol* 1988;17:248–54.

184. Fox AJ, Collier PF. Low mortality rates in industrial cohort studies due to selection for work and survival in the industry. *Br J Prev Soc Med* 1976;30:225–30.

185. Fox JP. Family-based epidemiologic studies. *Am J Epidemiol* 1974;99:165–79.

186. Frank JW. Causation revisited. *J Clin Epidemiol* 1988;41:425–6.
187. Fraser DW. Epidemiology as a liberal art. *N Engl J Med* 1987;316: 309–14.
188. Freeman J, Hutchinson GB. Prevalence, incidence and duration. *Am J Epidemiol* 1980;112:707–23.
189. Freeman J, Hutchinson GB. Duration of disease, duration indicators, and estimation of the risk ratio. *Am J Epidemiol* 1986;124:134–49.
190. Freeman RW, Bleecker ML, Comstock GW, Brookmeyer RS. Validation of self-administered questionnaire for study of peripheral neuropathy. *Am J Epidemiol* 1985;121:291–300.
191. Freiman JA, Chalmers TC, Smith H, Kuebler RR. The importance of beta, the Type II error and sample size in the design and interpretation of the randomized control trial. Survey of 71 "negative" trials. *N Engl J Med* 1978;299:690–4.
192. Freudenheim JL, Johnson NE, Wardrop RL. Misclassification of nutrient intake of individuals and groups using one-, two-, three-, and seven-day food records. *Am J Epidemiol* 1987;126:703–13.
193. Freudenheim JL, Johnson NE, Wardrop RL. Nutrient misclassification: bias in the odds ratio and loss of power in the Mantel test for trend. *Int J Epidemiol* 1989;18:232–8.
194. Fried LP, Pearson TA. The association of risk factors with arteriographically defined coronary artery disease: what is the appropriate control group? *Am J Epidemiol* 1987;125:844–53.
195. Friedman LM, Furberg CO, DeMets DL. Fundamentals of clinical trials (second edition). PSG Publishing Company Inc, Littleton 1985.
196. Friend JW, Feibleman J. What science really means. An explanation of the history and empirical method of general science. George Allen & Unwin Ltd, London 1937.
197. Froggatt P. Determinants of policy on smoking and health. *Int J Epidemiol* 1989;18:1–9.
198. Frost F, Jennings T, Starzyk P. Completeness of infant death registration for very low birthweight infants: Washington State 1978-79. *Am J Pub Health* 1982;72:740–1.
199. Fung KY, Howe GR. Methodological issues in case-control studies III: the effect of joint misclassification of risk factors and confounding factors upon estimation and power. *Int J Epidemiol* 1984;13:366–70.
200. Gamble J, Spirtas R. Job classification and utilization of complete work histories in occupational epidemiology. *J Occup Med* 1976;18: 399–404.
201. Garfield E. How we evaluate the health risks of toxic substances in the environment. Current Contents, August 20, 1982:5–11.
202. Gerbarg ZB, Horwitz RI. Resolving conflicting clinical trials: guidelines for meta-analysis. *J Clin Epidemiol* 1988;41:503–9.
203. Gillick MR. Common-sense models of health and disease. *N Engl J Med* 1985;313:700–3.
204. Gjorup T, Bugge PM, Hendriksen C, Jensen AM. A critical evaluation of the clinical diagnosis of anemia. *Am J Epidemiol* 1986;124:657–65.
205. Gladen B, Rogan WJ. Misclassification and the design of environmental studies. *Am J Epidemiol* 1979;109:607–16.

206. Goldberger J, Waring CH, Willets DG. The treatment and prevention of pellagra. *Public Health Rep* 1914;29:2821-5.
207. Goldberger J, Wheeler GA, Lillie RD, Rogers LM. A further study of butter, fresh beef, and yeast as pellagra preventives, with consideration of the relation of factor P of pellagra (and black tongue of dogs) to vitamin B. *Public Health Rep* 1926;41:297-318.
208. Goldsmith JR. Epidemiology and environmental health policy. *Int J Epidemiol* 1972;1:93-100.
209. Goodman SN, Royall R. Evidence and scientific research. *Am J Pub Health* 1988;78:1568-74.
210. Gordis L. Should dead cases be matched to dead controls? *Am J Epidemiol* 1982;115:1-5.
211. Gordis L. Challenges to epidemiology in the next decade. *Am J Epidemiol* 1988;128:1-9.
212. Gordis L, Gold E, Seltser R. Privacy protection in epidemiologic and medical research: a challenge and a responsibility. *Am J Epidemiol* 1977;105:163-8.
213. Gordon T, Sorlie P, Kannel WB. Problems in the assessment of blood pressure: the Framingham study. *Int J Epidemiol* 1976;5:327-34.
214. Graham S. Enhancing creativity in epidemiology. *Am J Epidemiol* 1988;128:249-53.
215. Graham S, Graham-Tomasi R. Achieved status as a risk factor in epidemiology. *Am J Epidemiol* 1985;122:553-8.
216. Gray-Donald K, Kramer MS. Causality inference in observational vs experimental studies. An empirical comparison. *Am J Epidemiol* 1988;127:885-92.
217. Grayson DA. Confounding confounding. *Am J Epidemiol* 1987; 126:546-53. The author replies. *Am J Epidemiol* 1989;129: 1089-91.
218. Green SB, Byar DP. The effect of stratified randomization on size and power of statistical tests in clinical trials. *J Chron Dis* 1978;31:445-54.
219. Greenberg BG. The future of epidemiology. *J Chron Dis* 1983;36: 353-9.
220. Greenberg ER, Rosner B, Hennekens C et al. An investigation of bias in a study of nuclear shipyard workers. *Am J Epidemiol* 1985;121: 301-8.
221. Greenfield S. The state of outcome research: are we on target? *N Engl J Med* 1989;320:1142-3.
222. Greenland S. Response and follow-up bias in cohort studies. *Am J Epidemiol* 1977;106:184-7.
223. Greenland S. The effect of misclassification in the presence of covariates. *Am J Epidemiol* 1980;112:564-9.
224. Greenland S. Interpretation and estimation of summary ratios under heterogeneity. *Stat Med* 1982a;1:217-27.
225. Greenland S. The effect of misclassification in matched-pair case-control studies. *Am J Epidemiol* 1982b;116:402-6.
226. Greenland S. A counterexample to the test-based principle of setting confidence limits. *Am J Epidemiol* 1984;120:4-7.
227. Greenland S. Control-initiated case-control studies. *Int J Epidemiol* 1985;14:130-4.

228. Greenland S. Identifiability, exchangeability and epidemiological confounding. *Int J Epidemiol* 1986a;15:412–8.
229. Greenland S. Cohorts versus dynamic populations: a dissenting view. *J Chron Dis* 1986b;39:565–6.
230. Greenland S. Interpretation and choice of effect measures in epidemiologic analyses. *Am J Epidemiol* 1987a;125:761–8.
231. Greenland S (ed). Evolution of epidemiologic ideas. Annotated readings on concepts and methods. Epidemiology Resources Inc, Chestnut Hill 1987b.
232. Greenland S. On sample-size and power calculations for studies using confidence intervals. *Am J Epidemiol* 1988a;128:231–7.
233. Greenland S. Statistical uncertainty due to misclassification: implications for validation substudies. *J Clin Epidemiol* 1988b;41:1167–74.
234. Greenland S, Freirichs RR. On measures and models for the effectiveness of vaccines and vaccination programmes. *Int J Epidemiol* 1988; 17:456–63.
235. Greenland S, Kleinbaum DG. Correcting for misclassification in two-way tables and matched-pair studies. *Int J Epidemiol* 1983; 12:93–7.
236. Greenland S, Morgenstern H. Classification schemes for epidemiologic research designs. *J Clin Epidemiol* 1988;41:715–6.
237. Greenland S, Morgenstern H. Ecological bias, confounding, and effect modification. *Int J Epidemiol* 1989a;18:269–74.
238. Greenland S, Morgenstern H. What is directionality? *J Clin Epidemiol* 1989b;42:821–4.
239. Greenland S, Morgenstern H, Poole C, Robins JM. Re: Confounding confounding. *Am J Epidemiol* 1989:129:1086–9.
240. Greenland S, Morgenstern H, Thomas DS. Considerations in determining matching criteria and stratum sizes for case-control studies. *Int J Epidemiol* 1981;10:389–92.
241. Greenland S, Neutra R. Control of confounding in the assessment of medical technology. *Int J Epidemiol* 1980;9:361–7.
242. Greenland S, Neutra R. An analysis of detection bias and proposed corrections in the study of estrogens and endometrial cancer. *J Chron Dis* 1981;34:433–8.
243. Greenland S, Robins JM. Confounding and misclassification. *Am J Epidemiol* 1985;122:495–506.
244. Greenland S, Robins JM. Identifiability, exchangeability, and epidemiological confounding. *Int J Epidemiol* 1986;15:413–9.
245. Greenland S, Robins JM. Conceptual problems in the definition and interpretation of attributable fractions. *Am J Epidemiol* 1988;128: 1185–97.
246. Greenland S, Thomas DC. On the need for the rare disease assumption in case-control studies. *Am J Epidemiol* 1982;116:547–53.
247. Greenland, S, Thomas DC, Morgenstern H. The rare-disease assumption revisited. A critique of "estimators of relative risk for case-control studies". *Am J Epidemiol* 1986;124:869–76.
248. Gullen WH, Bearman JE, Johnson EA. Effects of misclassification in epidemiologic studies. *Public Health Rep* 1968;83:914–8.

249. Guyatt GH, Townsend M, Keller JL, Singer J. Should study subjects see their previous responses: data from a randomized control trial. *J Clin Epidemiol* 1989;42:913–20.

250. Guyatt G, Walter S, Norman G. Measuring change over time: assessing the usefulness of evaluative instruments. *J Chron Dis* 1987; 40:171–8.

251. Haley NJ, Axelrad CM, Tilton KA. Validation of self-reported smoking behavior: biochemical analyses of cotinine and thiocyanate. *Am J Pub Health* 1983;73:1204–7.

252. Haley RW, Schaberg DR, McClish DK et al. The accuracy of retrospective chart review in measuring nosocomial infection rates. Results of validation studies in pilot hospitals. *Am J Epidemiol* 1980;111: 516–33.

253. Harlow BL, Davis S. Two one-step methods for household screening and interviewing using random digit dialing. *Am J Epidemiol* 1988; 127:857–63.

254. Harlow SD, Linet MS. Agreement between questionnaire data and medical records. *Am J Epidemiol* 1989;129:233–48.

255. Harter L, Starzyk P, Frost F. A comparative study of hospital fetal death records and Washington State fetal death certificates. *Am J Pub Health* 1986;76:1333–4.

256. Hartge P, Cahill JI, West D et al. Design and methods in a multi-center case-control interview study. *Am J Pub Health* 1984;74:52–6.

257. Heederik D, Miller BG. Weak associations in occupational epidemiology: adjustment for exposure estimation error. *Int J Epidemiol* 1988;17:970–4.

258. Helsing KJ, Comstock GW. Response variation and location of questions within a questionnaire. *Int J Epidemiol* 1976;5:125–30.

259. Hemminki E, Rahkonen O, Rimpalë M. Selection to coffee drinking by health—who becomes an adolescent coffee drinker? *Am J Epidemiol* 1988;127:1088–90.

260. Hennessy TW, Ballard DJ, DeRemee RA et al. The influence of diagnostic access bias on the epidemiology of sarcoidosis: a population-based study in Rochester, Minnesota, 1935-1984. *J Clin Epidemiol* 1988;41:565–70.

261. Herrman N. Retrospective information from questionnaires. I. Comparability of primary respondents and their next-of-kin. *Am J Epidemiol* 1985a;121:937–47.

262. Herrman N. Retrospective information from questionnaires. II. Intrarater reliability and comparison of questionnaire types. *Am J Epidemiol* 1985b;121:948–53.

263. Hertzman C. Evidence of a pitfall in control selection for a community-based environment health survey. *Am J Epidemiol* 1988; 127:407–10.

264. Hertzman C, Walter SD, From L, Alison A. Observer perception of skin color in a study of malignant melanoma. *Am J Epidemiol* 1987;126:901–11.

265. Higginson J. Publication of "negative" epidemiological studies. *J Chron Dis* 1987;40:371–2.

266. Hill AB. Observation and experiment. *N Engl J Med* 1953;248: 995–1001.
267. Hill AB. The environment and disease: association or causation? *Proc R Soc Med* 1965;58:295–300.
268. Hill P, Haley NJ, Wynder EL. Cigarette smoking: carboxyhemoglobin, plasma nicotine, cotinine and thiocyanate vs self-reported smoking data and cardiovascular disease. *J Chron Dis* 1983;36: 439–49.
269. Hlatky MA, Mark DB, Califf RM, Pryor DB. Angina, myocardial ischemia and coronary disease: gold standards, operational definitions and correlations. *J Clin Epidemiol* 1989;42:381–4.
270. Hoar SK, Morrison AS, Cole P, Silverman DT. An occupation and exposure linkage system for the study of occupational carcinogenesis. *J Occup Med* 1980;22:722–6.
271. Hogan MD, Kupper LL, Most BM, Haseman JK. Alternatives to Rothman's approach for assessing synergism (or antagonism) in cohort studies. *Am J Epidemiol* 1978;108:60–7.
272. Hogue CJR, Gaylor DW, Schulz KF. The case-exposure study. A further explication and response to a critique. *Am J Epidemiol* 1986;124:877–83.
273. Hornsby PP, Wilcox AJ. Validity of questionnaire information on frequency of coitus. *Am J Epidemiol* 1989;130:94–9.
274. Horst CH, Obermann-de Boer GL, Kromhout D. Validity of the 24-hour recall method in infancy: the Leiden pre-school children study. *Int J Epidemiol* 1988;17:217–21.
275. Horwitz O, Lysgaard-Hansen B. Medical observations and bias. *Am J Epidemiol* 1975;101:391–9.
276. Horwitz RI. Comparison of epidemiologic data from multiple sources. *J Chron Dis* 1986;39:889–96.
277. Horwitz RI. The experimental paradigm and observational studies of cause-effect relationships in clinical medicine. *J Chron Dis* 1987; 40:91–9.
278. Horwitz RI, Feinstein AR. Alternative analytic methods for case-control studies of estrogens and endometrial cancer. *N Engl J Med* 1978;299:1089–94.
279. Horwitz RI, Feinstein AR, Horwitz SM, Robboy SJ. Necropsy diagnosis of endometrial cancer and detection-bias in case/control studies. *Lancet* 1981;2:66–8.
280. Horwitz RI, Yu EC. Problems and proposals for interview data in epidemiological research. *Int J Epidemiol* 1985;14:463–7.
281. House AE. Detecting bias in observational data. *Behav Assess* 1980; 231:29–31.
282. Howe GR. Methodological issues in cohort studies: point estimators of the rate ratio. *Int J Epidemiol* 1986;15:257–62.
283. Howe GR, Chiarelli AM, Lindsay JP. Components and modifiers of the healthy worker effect: evidence from three occupational cohorts and implications for industrial compensation *Am J Epidemiol* 1988;128:1364–75.
284. Howe GR, Choi BCK. Methodological issues in case-control studies:

validity and power of various design/analysis strategies. *Int J Epidemiol* 1983;12:238–45.

285. Howe GR, Harrison L, Jain M. A short diet history for assessing dietary exposure to N-Nitrosamines in epidemiologic studies. *Am J Epidemiol* 1986;124:595–601.

286. Hulka BS, Grimson RC, Greenberg BG et al. "Alternative" controls in a case-control study of endometrial cancer and exogenous estrogen. *Am J Epidemiol* 1980;112:376–87.

287. Hulka BS, Hogue CJR, Greenberg BG. Methodological issues in epidemiologic studies of endometrial cancer and exogenous estrogen. *Am J Epidemiol* 1978;107:267–76.

288. Hulley SB. Symposium on CHD prevention trials: design issues in testing life style intervention. *Am J Epidemiol* 1978;108:85–6.

289. Humble CG, Samet JM, Skipper BE. Comparison of self- and surrogate-reported dietary information. *Am J Epidemiol* 1984;119: 86–98.

290. Humble CG, Samet JM, Skipper BE. Use of quantified and frequency indices of vitamin A intake in a case-control study of lung cancer. *Int J Epidemiol* 1987;16:341–6.

291. Huncharek M. Re: Challenges to epidemiology in the next decade. *Am J Epidemiol* 1989;129:861.

292. Hunter DJ, Sampson L, Stampfer MJ et al. Variability in portion sizes of commonly consumed foods among a population of women in the United States. *Am J Epidemiol* 1988;127:1240–9.

293. Hutchinson GB, Rothman KJ. Correcting a bias? *N Engl J Med* 1978;299:1129–30.

294. Hutchinson TA, Lane DA. Standardized methods of causality assessment for suspected adverse drug reactions. *J Chron Dis* 1986; 39:857–60.

295. Hutchinson TA, Lane DA. Assessing methods for causality assessment of suspected adverse drug reactions. *J Clin Epidemiol* 1989;42:5–16.

296. Ibrahim MA, Spitzer WO. The case-control study: consensus and controversy. Pergamon Press, Oxford 1979.

297. Ingham JG, McC Miller P. The concept of prevalence applied to psychiatric disorders and symptoms. *Psychol Med* 1976;6:217–25.

298. Israel RA, Rosenberg HM, Curtin LR. Analytical potential for multiple cause-of-death data. *Am J Epidemiol* 1986;124:161–79.

299. Jackson R, Beaglehole R. Secular trends in underreporting of cigarette consumption. *Am J Epidemiol* 1985;122:341–4.

300. Jacobsen BK, Knutsen SF, Knutsen R. The Tromso heart study: comparison of information from a short food frequency questionnaire with a dietary history survey. *Scand J Soc Med* 1987;15:41–7.

301. Jacobsen M. Against Popperized epidemiology. *Int J Epidemiol* 1976;5:9–11.

302. Jain M. Howe GR, Harrison L, Miller AB. A study of repeatability of dietary data over a seven-year period. *Am J Epidemiol* 1989;129: 422–9.

303. Jain M, Howe GR, Johnson KC, Miller AB. Evaluation of a diet

history questionnaire for epidemiologic studies. *Am J Epidemiol* 1980;111:212–9.

304. Jarvis MJ, Tunstall-Pedoe H, Feyerabend C et al. Comparison of tests used to distinguish smokers from nonsmokers. *Am J Pub Health* 1987;77:1435–8.

305. Jick H, Vessey MP. Case-control studies in the evaluation of drug-induced illness. *Am J Epidemiol* 1978;107:1–7.

306. Johnston DW, Shaper AG. Type A behaviour in British men: reliability and intercorrelation of two measures. *J Chron Dis* 1983;36: 203–7.

307. Joint committee on governmental affairs of the epidemiology section (American Public Health Association) and the Society for Epidemiologic Research. Commentary: The interagency regulatory liaison group "guidelines for documentation of epidemiologic studies". *Am J Epidemiol* 1981;114:614–8.

308. Järvholm B. Comparing mortality in an occupational cohort with incidence rates of the general population—the bias introduced through the use of five-year age intervals. *Am J Epidemiol* 1987; 125:747–9.

309. Karhausen LR. Re: On the logic of causal inference. *Am J Epidemiol* 1987;126:556–7.

310. Karon JM, Kupper LL. In defense of matching. *Am J Epidemiol* 1982;116:852–66.

311. Kasl SV. Mortality and the business cycle: some questions about research strategies when utilizing macro-social and ecological data. *Am J Pub Health* 1979;69:784–8.

312. Kelsey JL, O'Brien LA, Grisso JA, Hoffman S. Issues in carrying out epidemiologic research in the elderly. *Am J Epidemiol* 1989;130: 857–66.

313. Kelson M, Farebrother M. The effect of inaccuracies in death certification and coding practices in the European Economic Community (EEC) on international cancer mortality statistics. *Int J Epidemiol* 1987;16:411–4.

314. Khosla T, Lowe CR. Indices of obesity derived from body weight and height. *Br J Prev Soc Med* 1967;21:122–8.

315. Khoury MJ, Beaty TH, Liang K-Y. Can familial aggregation of disease be explained by familial aggregation of environmental risk factors? *Am J Epidemiol* 1988;127:674–83.

316. Khoury MJ, Cohen BH. Concepts and terms in genetic epidemiology: some similarities to infectious disease epidemiology. *J Clin Epidemiol* 1988;41:1181–7.

317. Khoury MJ, Flanders WD, Greenland S, Adams MJ. On the measurement of susceptibility in epidemiologic studies. *Am J Epidemiol* 1989;129:183–90.

318. Khoury MJ, Flanders WD, James LM, Erickson JD. Human teratogens, prenatal mortality, and selection bias. *Am J Epidemiol* 1989; 130:361–70.

319. Khoury MJ, Stewart W, Beaty TH. The effect of genetic susceptibility

on causal inference in epidemiologic studies. *Am J Epidemiol* 1987;
126:561–7.

320. King ME, Soskolne CL. Use of modeling in infectious disease epidemiology. *Am J Epidemiol* 1988;128:949–61.

321. Kircher T, Nelson J, Burdo H. The autopsy as a measure of accuracy of the death certificate. *N Engl J Med* 1985;313:1263–9.

322. Kirscht JP. Social and psychological problems of surveys on health and illness. *Soc Sci Med* 71;5:519–26.

323. Klein R, Klein BEK, Moss SE, DeMets DL. The validity of a survey question to study diabetic retinopathy. *Am J Epidemiol* 1986;124:104–10.

324. Kleinbaum DG, Kupper LL, Morgenstern H. Epidemiologic research. Principles and quantitative methods. Van Nostrand Reinhold Co, New York 1982.

325. Kleinbaum DG, Morgenstern H, Kupper LL. Selection bias in epidemiologic studies. *Am J Epidemiol* 1981;113:452–63.

326. Knottnerus JA. Subject selection in hospital-based case-control studies. *J Chron Dis* 1987;40:183–5.

327. Kohl HW, Blair SN, Paffenbarger RS Jr et al. A mail survey of physical activity habits as related to measured physical fitness. *Am J Epidemiol* 1988;127:1228–39.

328. Kolonel LN, Hirohata T, Nomura AMY. Adequacy of survey data collected from substitute respondents. *Am J Epidemiol* 1977;106:476–84.

329. Koopman JS. Causal models and sources of interaction. *Am J Epidemiol* 1977;106:439–44.

330. Koopman JS. Interaction between discrete causes. *Am J Epidemiol* 1981;113:716–24.

331. Koran LM. The reliability of clinical methods, data and judgments I. *N Engl J Med* 1975a;293:642–6.

332. Koran LM. The reliability of clinical methods, data and judgments II. *N Engl J Med* 1975b;293:695–701.

333. Krall EA, Valadian I, Dwyer JT, Gardner J. Recall of childhood illnesses. *J Clin Epidemiol* 1988;41:1059–64.

334. Krall EA, Valadian I, Dwyer JT, Gardner J. Accuracy of recalled smoking data. *Am J Pub Health* 1989;79:200–2.

335. Kramer MS, Boivin J-F. Toward an "unconfounded" classification of epidemiologic research design. *J Chron Dis* 1987;40:683–8.

336. Kramer MS, Boivin J-F. The importance of directionality in epidemiologic research design. *J Clin Epidemiol* 1988;41:717–8. Response. 806.

337. Kramer MS, Boivin J-F. Directionality, timing, and sample selection in epidemiologic research design. *J Clin Epidemiol* 1989;42:827–8.

338. Krieger N. Re: On the logic of causal inference. *Am J Epidemiol* 1987;126:155–7.

339. Kuller LH. Epidemiology and health policy. *Am J Epidemiol* 1988;127:2–16.

340. Kupper LL. Effects of the use of unreliable surrogate variables on the

validity of epidemiologic research studies. *Am J Epidemiol* 1984; 120:643–8.

341. Kupper LL, Hogan MD. Interaction in epidemiologic studies. *Am J Epidemiol* 1978;108:447–53.

342. Kurland LT, Molgaard CA. The patient record in epidemiology. *Sci Am* 1981;245:46–55.

343. Kushi LH, Kaye SA, Folsom AR et al. Accuracy and reliability of self-measurement of body girths. *Am J Epidemiol* 1988;128:740–8.

343a.Lakatos I. Falsification and the methodology of scientific research programs. In: Lakatos I, Musgrave A (eds). Criticism and the growth of knowledge. Cambridge University Press, London 1984.

343b.Lanes S. The logic of causal inference. In: Rothman KJ (ed). Causal inference. Epidemiology Resources Inc., Chestnut Hill 1988.

343c.Lanes S. Error and uncertainty in causal inference. In: Rothman KJ (ed). Causal inference. Epidemiology Resources Inc., Chestnut Hill 1988.

344. Lanes SF, Poole C. "Truth in packaging?" The unwrapping of epidemiologic research. *J Occup Med* 1984;26:571–4.

345. Langmuir AD. William Farr: founder of modern concepts of surveillance. *Int J Epidemiol* 1976;5:13–8.

346. Last JM. Towards a dictionary of epidemiological terms. *Int J Epidemiol* 1982;11:188–9.

347. Last JM (ed). A dictionary of epidemiology (second edition). Oxford University Press, Oxford 1988.

348. Lawrence CE, Greenwald P. Epidemiologic screening: a method to add efficiency to epidemiologic research. *Am J Epidemiol* 1977;105: 575–81.

349. Leaderer BP, Zagraniski RT, Berwick M, Stolwijk JAJ. Assessment of exposure to indoor air contaminants from combustion sources: methodology and application. *Am J Epidemiol* 1986;124:275–89.

350. Lee J, Kolonel LN. Nutrient intakes of husbands and wives: implications for epidemiologic research. *Am J Epidemiol* 1982;115:515–25.

351. Lee-Feldstein, A. A comparison of several measures of exposure to arsenic. Matched case-control study of copper smelter employees. *Am J Epidemiol* 1989;129:112–24.

352. Lee-Han H, McGuire V, Boyd NF. A review of the methods used by studies of dietary measurement. *J Clin Epidemiol* 1989;42:269–79.

353. le Marchand L, Yoshizawa CN, Nomura AMY. Validation of body size information on driver's licenses. *Am J Epidemiol* 1988;128: 874–7.

354. Lemasters GK, Pinney SM. Employment status as a confounder when assessing occupational exposures and spontaneous abortion. *J Clin Epidemiol* 1989;42:975–81.

355. Lerchen ML, Samet JM. An assessment of the validity of questionnaire responses provided by a surviving spouse. *Am J Epidemiol* 1986;123:481–9.

356. Lerman SJ, Lerman LM, Nankervis GA, Gold E. Accuracy of rubella history. *Ann Int Med* 1971;74:97–8.

357. Levav I, Arnon A, Portnoy A. Two shortened versions of the Cornell

medical index—a new test of their validity. *Int J Epidemiol* 1977;6: 135–41.

358. Lichtenstein MJ, Mulrow CD, Elwood PC. Guidelines for reading case-control studies. *J Chron Dis* 1987;40:893–903.

359. Liddell FDK. The development of cohort studies in epidemiology: a review. *J Clin Epidemiol* 1988;41:1217–37.

360. Lilienfeld AM. Epidemiology of infectious and non-infectious disease: some comparisons. *Am J Epidemiol* 1973;97:135–47.

361. Lilienfeld AM. The surgeon general's "epidemiologic criteria for causality": a criticism of Burch's critique. *J Chron Dis* 1983;36: 837–45.

362. Lilienfeld AM, Lilienfeld DE. What else is new? An historical excursion. *Am J Epidemiol* 1977;105:169–79.

363. Lilienfeld DE. Definitions of epidemiology. *Am J Epidemiol* 1978; 107:87–90.

364. Lilienfeld DE, Lilienfeld AM. Epidemiology: a retrospective study. *Am J Epidemiol* 1977;106:445–59.

365. Linden G, Austin DF. A rapid reporting cancer incidence system. *Am J Epidemiol* 1974;99:180–1.

366. Linet MS, Brookmeyer R. Use of cancer controls in case-control cancer studies. *Am J Epidemiol* 1987;125:1–11.

367. Liu K. Measurement error and its impact on partial correlation and multiple linear regression analyses. *Am J Epidemiol* 1988;127: 864–74.

368. Liu K, Stamler J, Stamler R et al. Methodological problems in characterizing an individual's plasma glucose level. *J Chron Dis* 1982; 35:475–85.

369. Lossos I, Israeli A, Zajicek G, Berry EM. Diagnosis deferred—the clinical spectrum of diagnostic uncertainty. *J Clin Epidemiol* 1989; 42:649–57.

370. Lower GM Jr, Kanarek MS. The mutation theory of chronic, noninfectious disease: relevance to epidemiologic theory. *Am J Epidemiol* 1982;115:803–17.

371. Lubin JH, Gail MH. Biased selection of controls for case-control analyses of cohort studies. *Biometrics* 1984;40:63–75.

372. Luepker RV, Pallonen UE, Murray DM, Pirie PL. Validity of telephone surveys in assessing cigarette smoking in young adults. *Am J Pub Health* 1989;79:202–4.

373. Lund E. The validity of different control groups in a case-control study. Oral contraceptive use and breast cancer in young women. *J Clin Epidemiol* 1989;42:987–93.

374. Lyon JL, Robison LM, Moser R Jr. Uncertainty in the diagnosis of histologically confirmed pancreatic cancer cases. *Int J Epidemiol* 1989;18:305–8.

375. Mackenzie SG, Lippman A. An investigation of report bias in a case-control study of pregnancy outcome. *Am J Epidemiol* 1989;129: 65–75.

376. Maclure M. Popperian refutation in epidemiology. *Am J Epidemiol* 1985;121:343–50.

377. Maclure M. On the logic and practice of epidemiology. *Am J Epidemiol* 1987;126:554.
378. MacMahon B, Pugh TF. Epidemiology, principles and methods. Little, Brown & Co, Boston 1970.
379. Maheux B, Legault C, Lambert J. Increasing response rates in physicians' mail surveys: an experimental study. *Am J Pub Health* 1989; 79:638–9.
380. Mantel N. Familial breast cancer and the awareness bias. *Am J Epidemiol* 1987;125:920.
381. Marchbanks PA, Peterson HB, Rubin GL et al. Research on infertility: definition makes a difference. *Am J Epidemiol* 1989;130:259–67.
382. Marchevsky N, Held JR, Garcia-Carrillo C. Probability of introducing diseases because of false negative test results. *Am J Epidemiol* 1989;130:611–4.
383. Margetts BM, Cade JE, Osmond C. Comparison of a food frequency questionnaire with a diet record. *Int J Epidemiol* 1989;18:868–73.
384. Marks GC, Habicht J-P, Mueller WH. Reliability, dependability, and precision of anthropometric measurements. The second national health and nutrition examination survey 1976–1980. *Am J Epidemiol* 1989;130:578–87.
385. Marmot M, Winkelstein W. Epidemiologic observations on intervention trials for prevention of coronary heart disease. *Am J Epidemiol* 1975;101:177–81.
386. Marshall J, Priore R, Haughey B et al. Spouse-subject interviews and the reliability of diet studies. *Am J Epidemiol* 1980;112:675–83.
387. Martin CA, Jamrozik K, Armstrong BK et al. An unjustified attack on "incidence"? *Am J Epidemiol* 1989;129:653–4.
388. Mascioli SR, Jacobs DR Jr, Kottke TE. Diagnostic criteria for hospitalized acute myocardial infarction: the Minnesota experience. *Int J Epidemiol* 1989;18:76–83.
389. Mattsson B. Completeness of registration in the Swedish cancer registry. The National Central Bureau of Statistics, Statistical reports, HS 1977.12, Stockholm, Sweden.
390. Mattsson B, Rutqvist LE, Wallgren A. Undernotification of diagnosed cancer cases to the Stockholm Cancer Registry. *Int J Epidemiol* 1985;14:64–9.
391. Mayes LC, Horwitz RI, Feinstein AR. A collection of 56 topics with contradictory results in case-control research. *Int J Epidemiol* 1988; 17:680–3.
392. Mazumdar S, Colbus DS, Townsend MC. Validation of hospital discharge diagnosis data for chronic obstructive pulmonary disease and other allied conditions. *Am J Pub Health* 1986;76:803–5.
393. McDowell I, Praught E. On the measurement of happiness. An examination of the Bradburn scale in the Canada health survey. *Am J Epidemiol* 1982;116:949–58.
394. McGilchrist CA, Hills LJ. Estimation of cumulative illness using cross-sectional data. *J Chron Dis* 1986;39:929–31.
395. McKennel AC. Bias in the reported incidence of smoking by children. *Int J Epidemiol* 1980;9:167–77.

396. McKeown-Eyssen GE, Yeung KS, Bright-See E. Assessment of past diet in epidemiologic studies. *Am J Epidemiol* 1986;124:94–103.
397. McLaughlin JK, Blot WJ, Mehl ES, Mandel JS. Problems in the use of dead controls in case-control studies. I. General results. *Am J Epidemiol* 1985a;121:131–9.
398. McLaughlin JK, Blot WJ, Mehl ES, Mandel JS. Problems in the use of dead controls in case-control studies. II. Effect of excluding certain causes of death. *Am J Epidemiol* 1985b;122:485–94.
399. McLaughlin JK, Dietz MS, Mehl ES, Blot WJ. Reliability of surrogate information on cigarette smoking by type of informant. *Am J Epidemiol* 1987;126:144–6.
400. McMichael AJ. Standardized mortality ratios and the "Healthy worker effect": scratching beneath the surface. *J Occup Med* 1976; 18:165–8.
401. McMichael AJ. Assigning handicaps in the mortality stakes: an evaluation of the "Healthy worker effect". Industrial Disease Standards Panel, Ontario Ministry of Labor;Sept 1987:1–14.
402. McMichael AJ. Setting environmental exposure standards: the role of the epidemiologist. *Int J Epidemiol* 1989;18:10–6.
403. McTiernan A, Thomas DB, Whitehead A, Noonan E. Efficient selection of controls for multi-centered collaborative studies of rare diseases. *Am J Epidemiol* 1986;123:901–4.
404. McTiernan A, Weiss NS, Daling JR. Bias resulting from using the card-back system to contact patients in an epidemiologic study. *Am J Pub Health* 1986;76:71–3.
405. Meltzer JW, Hochstim JR. Reliability and validity of survey data on physical health. *Public Health Rep* 1970;85:1075–86.
406. Meydrech EF, Kupper LL. Cost considerations and sample size requirements in cohort and case-control studies. *Am J Epidemiol* 1978;107:201–5.
407. Mickey RM, Greenland S. The impact of confounder selection criteria on effect estimation. *Am J Epidemiol* 1989;129:125–37.
408. Miettinen OS. Individual matching with multiple controls in the case of all-or-none responses. *Biometrics* 1969;25:339–55.
409. Miettinen OS. Matching and design efficiency in retrospective studies. *Am J Epidemiol* 1970;91:111-8.
410. Miettinen OS. Components of the crude risk ratio. *Am J Epidemiol* 1972;96:168–72.
411. Miettinen OS. Proportion of disease caused or prevented by a given exposure, trait or intervention. *AM J Epidemiol* 1974a;99:325–32.
412. Miettinen OS. Confounding and effect modification. *Am J Epidemiol* 1974b;100:350–3.
413. Miettinen OS. Estimability and estimation in case-referent studies. *Am J Epidemiol* 1976a;103:226–35.
414. Miettinen OS. Stratification by a multivariate confounder score. *Am J Epidemiol* 1976b;104:609–20.
415. Miettinen OS. Causal and preventive interdependence. Elementary principles. *Scand J Work Environ Health* 1982a;8:159–68.

416. Miettinen OS. Design options in epidemiologic research. An update. *Scand J Work Environ Health* 1982b;8(suppl 1):7–14.
417. Miettinen OS. The need for randomization in the study of intended effects. *Stat Med* 1983;2:267–71.
418. Miettinen OS. Theoretical epidemiology. Principles of occurrence research in medicine. John Wiley & Sons, New York 1985a.
419. Miettinen OS. The "case-control" study: valid selection of subjects. *J Chron Dis* 1985b;38:543–8. Author's response. *J Chron Dis* 1985c;38:557–8. Response. *J Chron Dis* 1986;39:567.
420. Miettinen OS. Subject selection in case-referent studies with a secondary base. *J Chron Dis* 1987;40:186–7.
421. Miettinen OS. Striving to deconfound the fundamentals of epidemiologic study design. *J Clin Epidemiol* 1988;41:709–13.
422. Miettinen OS. The clinical trial as a paradigm for epidemiologic research. *J Clin Epidemiol* 1989a;42:491–6.
423. Miettinen OS. Unlearned lessons from clinical trials: a duality of outlooks. *J Clin Epidemiol* 1989b;42:499–502.
424. Miettinen OS. "Directionality" in epidemiologic research. *J Clin Epidemiol* 1989c;42:825–6.
425. Miettinen OS, Caro JJ. Principles of nonexperimental assessment of excess risk, with special reference to adverse drug reactions. *J Clin Epidemiol* 1989;42:325–31.
426. Miettinen OS, Cook EF. Confounding: essence and detection. *Am J Epidemiol* 1981;114:593–603.
427. Miettinen OS, Wang J-D. An alternative to the proportionate mortality ratio. *Am J Epidemiol* 1981;114:144–8.
428. Miller AB. Hospital or population controls, an unanswered question. *J Chron Dis* 1984;37:337–8.
429. Miller TQ, Turner CW, Tindale RS, Posavac EJ. Disease based spectrum bias in referred samples and the relationship between type A behavior and coronary artery disease. *J Clin Epidemiol* 1988;41:1139–49.
430. Mitchell AA, Cottler LB, Shapiro S. Effect of questionnaire design on recall of drug exposure in pregnancy. *Am J Epidemiol* 1986;123:670–6.
431. Moens GFG. The reliability of reported suicide mortality statistics: an experience from Belgium. *Int J Epidemiol* 1985;14:272–5.
432. Monson RR. Occupational epidemiology. CRC Press Inc, Boca Raton 1980.
433. Morgan KJ, Johnson SR, Goungetas B. Variability of food intakes: an analysis of a 12-day data series using persistence measures. *Am J Epidemiol* 1987;126:326–35.
434. Morgan RW, Jain M, Miller AB et al. A comparison of dietary methods in epidemiologic studies. *Am J Epidemiol* 1978;107:488–98.
435. Morgenstern H. Uses of ecologic analysis in epidemiologic research. *Am J Pub Health* 1982;72:1336–44.
436. Morgenstern H, Kleinbaum DG, Kupper LL. Measures of disease

incidence used in epidemiologic research. *Int J Epidemiol* 1980;9: 97–104.

437. Morgenstern H, Winn DM. A method for determining the sampling ratio in epidemiologic studies. *Stat Med* 1983;2:387–96.
438. Morrison AS. Sequential pathogenic components of rates. *Am J Epidemiol* 1979;109:709–18.
439. Morrison AS. Case definition in case-control studies of the efficacy of screening. *Am J Epidemiol* 1982;115:6–8.
440. Moyer LA, Boyle CA, Pollock DA. Validity of death certificates for injury-related causes of death. *Am J Epidemiol* 1989;130:1024–32.
441. Mueller BA, McTiernan A, Daling JR. Level of response in epidemiologic studies using the card-back system to contact subjects. *Am J Pub Health* 1986;76:1331–2.
442. Mulder PGH, Garretsen HFL. Are epidemiological and sociological surveys a proper instrument for detecting true problem drinkers? (The low sensitivity of an alcohol survey in Rotterdam). *Int J Epidemiol* 1983;12:442–4.
443. Mullooly JP. Sample sizes for estimation of exposure-specific disease rates in population-based case-control studies. *Am J Epidemiol* 1987;125:1079–84.
444. Mulvihill JJ, Tulinius H. Cancer ecogenetics: studying genetic and environment interactions through epidemiology. *Int J Epidemiol* 1987;16:337–40.
445. Murphy EA. The normal. *Am J Epidemiol* 1973;98:403–11.
446. Murphy EA. The basis for interpreting family history. *Am J Epidemiol* 1989;129:19–22.
447. Moller Jensen O, Mosbech J, Salaspuro M, Jhamäki T. A comparative study of the diagnostic basis for cancer of the colon and cancer of the rectum in Denmark and Finland. *Int J Epidemiol* 1974;3:183–6.
448. Moller Jensen O, Wahrendorf J, Rosenqvist A, Geser A. The reliability of questionnaire-derived historical dietary information and temporal stability of food habits in individuals. *Am J Epidemiol* 1984;120:281–90.
449. Nelson LM, Franklin GM, Hamman RF et al. Referral bias in multiple sclerosis research. *J Clin Epidemiol* 1988;41:187–92.
450. Neuberger JS, Cuppage FE. Re: Methods of cancer case selection: implications for research. *Am J Epidemiol* 1985;121:324.
451. Newland CA, Waters WE, Standford AP, Batchelor BG. A study of mail survey method. *Int J Epidemiol* 1977;6:65–7.
452. Newman TB, Browner WS. The epidemiology of life and death: a critical commentary. *Am J Pub Health* 1988;78:161–2.
453. Norell SE. Accuracy of patient interviews and estimates by clinical staff in determining medication compliance. *Soc Sci Med* 1981; 15E:57–61.
454. Norell SE, Ahlbom A. Hospital vs population referents in two case-referent studies. *Scand J Work Environ Health* 1987;13:62–6.
455. Nurminen M. Some remarks on the operation of biases. *Scand J Work Environ Health* 1983;9:377–83.
456. Oakes TW, Friedman GD, Seltzer CC. Mail survey responses by

health status of smokers, nonsmokers, and ex-smokers. *Am J Epidemiol* 1973;98:50–5.

457. Oalmann MC, McGill HC Jr, Deupree RH. Cardiovascular mortality in a community: methodology and objective diagnostic criteria. *Am J Epidemiol* 1971;94:531–45.

458. Olsen GW, Mandel JS. Selection of elderly controls using random digit dialing. *Am J Pub Health* 1988;78:1487–8.

459. O'Neill RT. Sample sizes for estimation of the odds ratio in unmatched case-control studies. *Am J Epidemiol* 1984;120:145–53.

460. O'Neill RT, Anello C. Case-control studies: a sequential approach. *Am J Epidemiol* 1978;108:415–24.

461. O'Rourke K, Detsky AS. Meta-analysis in medical research: strong encouragement for higher quality in individual research efforts. *J Clin Epidemiol* 1989;42:1021–4.

462. Osmond C, Gardner MJ. Age, period, and cohort models. Nonoverlapping cohorts don't resolve the identification problem. *Am J Epidemiol* 1989;129:31–5.

463. O'Toole BI, Battistutta D, Long A, Crouch K. A comparison of costs and data quality of three health survey methods: mail, telephone and personal home interview. *Am J Epidemiol* 1986;124:317–28.

464. Paganini-Hill A, Ross RK. Reliability of recall of drug usage and other health-related information. *Am J Epidemiol* 1982;116:114–22.

465. Palta M, Prineas RJ, Berman R, Hannan P. Comparison of self-reported and measured height and weight. *Am J Epidemiol* 1982; 115:223–30.

466. Pasternack BS, Shore RE. Sample sizes for group sequential cohort and case-control study designs. *Am J Epidemiol* 1981;113:182–91.

467. Pastides H, Calabrese EJ, Hosmer DW, Harris DR. Validation of work histories obtained from interviews. *Am J Epidemiol* 1989;129:640–1.

468. Patriarca PA, Biellik RJ, Sanden G et al. Sensitivity and specificity of clinical case definitions for pertussis. *Am J Pub Health* 1988;78: 833–6.

469. Peace KE. The alternative hypothesis: one-sided or two-sided? *J Clin Epidemiol* 1989;42:473–6.

470. Pearce N, Checkoway H. Case-control studies using other diseases as controls: problems of excluding exposure-related diseases. *Am J Epidemiol* 1988;127:851–6.

471. Pearce N, Checkoway H, Shy C. Time-related factors as potential confounders and effect modifiers in studies based on an occupational cohort. *Scand J Work Environ Health* 1986;12:97–107.

472. Pearce N, Crawford-Brown D. Critical discussion in epidemiology: problems with the Popperian approach. *J Clin Epidemiol* 1989;42: 177–84.

473. Pecoraro RE, Inui TS, Chen MS et al. Validity and reliability of a self-administered health history questionnaire. *Public Health Rep* 1979; 94:231–8.

474. Percy C, Muir C. The international comparability of cancer mortality data. Results of an international death certificate study. *Am J Epidemiol* 1989;129:934–46.

475. Perkoff GT. The virtue of unconventional research. *J Clin Epidemiol* 1989;42:281–7.
476. Pershagen G, Axelson O. Validation of questionnaire information on occupational exposure and smoking. *Scand J Work Environ Health* 1982;8:24–8.
477. Persson I, Bergkvist L, Adami H-O. Reliability of women's histories of climacteric oestrogen treatment assessed by prescription forms. *Int J Epidemiol* 1987;16:222–8.
478. Persson LÅ, Carlgren G. Measuring children's diets: evaluation of dietary assessment techniques in infancy and childhood. *Int J Epidemiol* 1984;13:506–17.
479. Persson P-G, Norell SE. Retrospective versus original information on cigarette smoking. Implications for epidemiologic studies. *Am J Epidemiol* 1989;130:705–12.
480. Petersen DJ, Alexander GR, Powell-Griner E, Tompkins ME. Variations in the reporting of gestational age at induced termination of pregnancy. *Am J Pub Health* 1989;79:603–6.
481. Petitti DB, Friedman GD, Kahn W. Accuracy of information on smoking habits provided on self-administered research questionnaires. *Am J Pub Health* 1981;71:308–11.
482. Peto R, Pike MC, Armitage P et al. Design and analysis of randomized clinical trials requiring prolonged observation of each patient. I. Introduction and design. *Br J Cancer* 1976;34:585–612.
483. Phillips AN, Pocock SJ. Sample size requirements for prospective studies, with examples for coronary heart disease. *J Clin Epidemiol* 1989;42:639–48.
484. Piantadosi S, Byar DP, Green SB. The ecological fallacy. *Am J Epidemiol* 1988;127:893–904.
485. Pickle LW, Brown LM, Blot WJ. Information available from surrogate respondents in case-control interview studies. *Am J Epidemiol* 1983; 118:99–108.
486. Pierce JP, Dwyer T, DiGiusto E et al. Cotinine validation of self-reported smoking in commercially run community surveys. *J Chron Dis* 1987;40:689–95.
487. Pietinen P, Hartman, Haapa E et al. Reproducibility and validity of dietary assessment instruments. I. A self-administered food use questionnaire with a portion size picture booklet. *Am J Epidemiol* 1988a;128:655–66.
488. Pietinen P, Hartman AM, Haapa E et al. Reproducibility and validity of dietary assessment instruments. II. A qualitative food frequency questionnaire. *Am J Epidemiol* 1988b;128:667–76.
489. Pike MC, Casagrande JT. Re: Cost considerations and sample size requirements in cohort and case-control studies. *Am J Epidemiol* 1979;110:100–2. Correction 1982;116:198.
490. Pike MC, Robins J. Re: Possibility of selection bias in matched case-control studies using friend controls. *Am J Epidemiol* 1989;130: 209–10.
491. Pocock SJ. Current issues in the design and interpretation of clinical trials. *Br Med J* 1985a;290:39–42.

492. Pocock SJ. Clinical trials—a practical approach. John Wiley and Sons, Chichester 1985b.

493. Poole C. Exposure opportunity in case-control studies. *Am J Epidemiol* 1986;123:352–8.

494. Poole C. Critical appraisal of the exposure-potential restriction rule. *Am J Epidemiol* 1987a;125:179–83.

495. Poole C. Beyond the confidence interval. *Am J Pub Health* 1987b; 77:195–9.

496. Poole C. Confidence intervals exclude nothing. *Am J Pub Health* 1987c;77:492–3.

497. Poole C. Feelings and frequencies: two kinds of probability in public health research. *Am J Pub Health* 1988;78:1531–2.

498. Popiela T, Jedrychowski W, Filipek A et al. Validity of questionnaire criteria in mass screening for the diagnosis of peptic ulcer. *Int J Epidemiol* 1976;5:251–3.

498a. Popper KR. Conjectures and refutations: the growth of scientific knowledge. Harper, New York 1963.

499. Preston SH. Relations among standard epidemiologic measures in a population. *Am J Epidemiol* 1987;126:336–45.

500. Preston-Martin S, Bernstein L, Maldonado AA et al. A dental X-ray validation study. Comparison of information from patient interviews and dental charts. *Am J Epidemiol* 1985;121:430–9.

501. Pron GE, Burch JD, Howe GR, Miller AB. The reliability of passive smoking histories reported in a case-control study of lung cancer. *Am J Epidemiol* 1988;127:267–73.

502. Prothero RM. Disease and mobility: a neglected factor in epidemiology. *Int J Epidemiol* 1977;6:259–67.

503. Quade D, Lachenbruch PA, Whaley FS et al. Effects of misclassification on statistical inferences in epidemiology. *Am J Epidemiol* 1980;111:503–15.

504. Ranstam J. Comparisons of standardized mortality ratios. *Scand J Work Environ Health* 1984;10:63.

505. Raphael K. Recall bias: a proposal for assessment and control. *Int J Epidemiol* 1987;16:167–70.

506. Ray WA, Griffin MR. Use of medicaid data for pharmacoepidemiology. *Am J Epidemiol* 1989;129:837–49.

507. Reger RB, Butcher DF, Morgan WKC. Assessing change in the pneumoconioses using serial radiographs. Sources and quantification of bias. *Am J Epidemiol* 1973;98:243–54.

508. Relman AS, Angell M. How good is peer review? *N Engl J Med* 1989;321:827–9.

509. Richardson S, Stücker I, Hémon D. Comparison of relative risks obtained in ecological and individual studies: some methodological considerations. *Int J Epidemiol* 1987;16:111–20.

510. Robins JM, Greenland S. The role of model selection in causal inference from nonexperimental data. *Am J Epidemiol* 1986;123:392–402.

511. Robinson H. Re: Causality inference in observational vs experimental studies: an empirical comparison. *Am J Epidemiol* 1989;130:206–8.

512. Robles SC, Marrett LD, Clarke EA, Risch HA. An application of capture-recapture methods to the estimation of completeness of cancer registration. *J Clin Epidemiol* 1988;41:495–501.

513. Rocca WA, Fratiglioni L, Bracco L et al. The use of surrogate respondents to obtain questionnaire data in case-control studies of neurologic diseases. *J Chron Dis* 1986;39:907–12.

514. Rogot E, Reid DD. The validity of data from next-of-kin in studies of mortality among migrants. *Int J Epidemiol* 1975;4:51–4.

515. Rohan TE, Potter JD. Retrospective assessment of dietary intake. *Am J Epidemiol* 1984;120:876–87.

516. Roidt L, White E, Goodman GE et al. Association of food frequency questionnaire estimates of vitamin A intake with serum vitamin A levels. *Am J Epidemiol* 1988;128:645–54.

517. Rolnick SJ, Gross CR, Garrard J, Gibson RW. A comparison of response rate, data quality, and cost in the collection of data on sexual history and personal behaviours. Mail survey approaches and in-person interview. *Am J Epidemiol* 1989;129:1052–61.

518. Roos LL Jr, Nicol JP, Cageorge SM. Using administrative data for longitudinal research: comparisons with primary data collection. *J Chron Dis* 1987;40:41–9.

519. Rose G. Sick individuals and sick populations. *Int J Epidemiol* 1985;14:32–8.

520. Rosenberg HM. Improving cause-of-death statistics. *Am J Pub Health* 1989;79:563–4.

521. Rosenberg L, Slone D, Shapiro S et al. Case-control studies on the acute effects of coffee upon the risk of myocardial infarction: problems in the selection of a hospital control series. *Am J Epidemiol* 1981;113:646–52.

522. Rosenberg MJ, Layde PM, Ory HW et al. Agreement between women's histories of oral contraceptive use and physician records. *Int J Epidemiol* 1983;12:84–7.

523. Rosner B, Cook NR, Evans DA et al. Reproducibility and predictive values of routine blood pressure measurements in children. Comparison with adult values and implications for screening children for elevated blood pressure. *Am J Epidemiol* 1987;126:1115–25.

524. Rosner B, Willett WC. Interval estimates for correlation coefficients corrected for within-person variation: implications for study design and hypothesis testing. *Am J Epidemiol* 1988;127:377–86.

525. Rothman KJ. Synergy and antagonism in cause-effect relationships. *Am J Epidemiol* 1974;99:385–8.

526. Rothman KJ. A pictorial representation of confounding in epidemiologic studies. *J Chron Dis* 1975;28:101–8.

527. Rothman KJ. Causes. *Am J Epidemiol* 1976a;104:587–92.

528. Rothman KJ. The estimation of synergy or antagonism. *Am J Epidemiol* 1976b;103:506–11.

529. Rothman KJ. Epidemiologic methods in clinical trials. *Cancer* 1977;39:1771–5.

530. Rothman KJ. Estimation versus detection in the assessment of synergy. *Am J Epidemiol* 1978a;108:9–11.

531. Rothman KJ. Occam's razor pares the choice among statistical models. *Am J Epidemiol* 1978b;108:347-9.

532. Rothman KJ. A show of confidence. *N Engl J Med* 1978c;299:1362-3.

533. Rothman KJ. Induction and latent periods. *Am J Epidemiol* 1981a; 114:253-9.

534. Rothman KJ. The rise and fall of epidemiology, 1950-2000 A.D. *N Engl J Med* 1981b;304:600-2.

535. Rothman KJ. Sleuthing in hospitals. *N Engl J Med* 1985;313:258-60.

536. Rothman KJ. Modern epidemiology. Little, Brown and Co, Boston 1986.

537. Rothman KJ. Clustering of disease. *Am J Pub Health* 1987;77:13-15.

538. Rothman KJ (ed). Causal inference. Epidemiology Resources Inc., Chestnut Hill 1988.

539. Rothman KJ, Greenland S, Walker AM. Concepts of interaction. *Am J Epidemiol* 1980;112:467-70.

540. Rothman KJ, Poole C. Science and policy making. *Am J Pub Health* 1985;75:340-1.

541. Rothman KJ, Poole C. A strengthening programme for weak associations. *Int J Epidemiol* 1988;17(suppl):955-9.

542. Rozman C, Marin P, Nomdedeu B, Montserrat E. Criteria for severe aplastic anaemia. *Lancet* 1987;2:955-7.

543. Russel-Briefel R, Caggiula AW, Kuller LH. A comparison of three dietary methods for estimating vitamin A intake. *Am J Epidemiol* 1985;122:628-36.

544. Sackett DL. Clinical epidemiology. *Am J Epidemiol* 1969;89:125-8.

545. Sackett DL. Bias in analytic research. *J Chron Dis* 1979;32:51-63.

546. Sackett DL. The competing objectives of randomized trials. *N Engl J Med* 1980;303:1059-60.

547. Sackett DL. Inference and decision at the bedside. *J Clin Epidemiol* 1989;42:309-16.

548. Sackett DL, Gent M. Controversy in counting and attributing events in clinical trials. *N Engl J Med* 1979;301:1410-2.

549. Sacks JJ, Krushat WM, Newman J. Reliability of the health hazard appraisal. *Am J Pub Health* 1980;70:730-2.

550. Saftlas AF, Satariano WA, Swanson GM et al. Methods of cancer case selection: implications for research. *Am J Epidemiol* 1983;118:852-6.

551. Salvini S, Hunter DJ, Sampson L et al. Food-based validation of a dietary questionnaire: the effects of week-to-week variation in food consumption. *Int J Epidemiol* 1989;18:858-67.

552. Samet JM. A historical and epidemiologic perspective on respiratory symptoms questionnaires. *Am J Epidemiol* 1978;108:435-46.

553. Samuels ML. Matching and design efficiency in epidemiological studies. *Biometrics* 1981;68:577-88.

554. Sandler DP, Shore DL. Quality of data on parent's smoking and drinking provided by adult offspring. *Am J Epidemiol* 1986;124: 768-78.

555. Saracci R. Interaction and synergism. *Am J Epidemiol* 1980;112: 465-6.

556. Sartwell PE. On the methodology of investigations of etiologic factors in chronic diseases—further comments. *J Chron Dis* 1960;11:61-3.

557. Sasco AJ. Lead time and length bias in case-control studies for the evaluation of screening. *J Clin Epidemiol* 1988;41:103–4.
558. Savitz DA, Barón AE. Estimating and correcting for confounder misclassification. *Am J Epidemiol* 1989;129:1062–71.
559. Savitz DA, Pearce N. Control selection with incomplete case ascertainment. *Am J Epidemiol* 1988;127:1109–17.
560. Saxén L, Klemetti A, Härö AS. A matched-pair register for studies of selected congenital defects. *Am J Epidemiol* 1974;100:297–306.
561. Schafer A. The ethics of the randomized clinical trial. *N Engl J Med* 1982;307:719–24.
562. Schatzkin A, Connor RJ, Taylor PR, Bunnag B. Comparing new and old screening tests when a reference procedure cannot be performed on all screenees. Example of automated cytometry for early detection of cervical cancer. *Am J Epidemiol* 1987;125:672–8.
563. Schatzkin A, Slud E. Competing risks bias arising from an omitted risk factor. *Am J Epidemiol* 1989;129:850–6.
564. Schlesselman JJ. Sample size requirements in cohort and case-control studies of disease. *Am J Epidemiol* 1974;99:381–4.
565. Schlesselman JJ. Assessing effects of confounding variables. *Am J Epidemiol* 1978;108:3–8.
566. Schlesselman JJ. Case-control studies. Design, conduct, analysis. Oxford University Press, New York 1982.
567. Schlesselman JJ. Valid selection of subjects in case-control studies. *J Chron Dis* 1985;38:549–50.
568. Schlesselman JJ. Re: Smallest detectable relative risk with multiple controls per case. *Am J Epidemiol* 1987;125:348.
569. Schlesselman JJ, Stadel BV. Exposure opportunity in epidemiologic studies. *Am J Epidemiol* 1987;125:174–8.
570. Schlesselman JJ, Stadel BV, Murray P et al. Consistency and plausibility in epidemiologic analysis: application to breast cancer in relation to use of oral contraceptives. *J Chron Dis* 1987;40:1033–9.
571. Schulte PA. Methodologic issues in the use of biologic markers in epidemiologic research. *Am J Epidemiol* 1987;126:1006–16.
572. Schulte PA, Ehrenberg RL, Singal M. Investigation of occupational cancer clusters: theory and practice. *Am J Pub Health* 1987;77:52–6.
573. Schulte PA, Singal M, Stringer WT et al. The efficacy of a population-based comparison group in cross-sectional occupational health studies. *Am J Epidemiol* 1982;116:981–9.
574. Schumacher MC. Comparison of occupation and industry information from death certificates and interviews. *Am J Pub Health* 1986; 76:635–7.
575. Schwartz GG. Re: On the logic of causal inference. *Am J Epidemiol* 1987;126:157.
576. Sears MR, Rea HH, de Boer G et al. Accuracy of certification of deaths due to asthma. *Am J Epidemiol* 1986;124:1004–11.
577. Seigel DG. The use of historical data and adverse reaction reporting systems for epidemiologic study. *Am J Epidemiol* 1971;94:210–4.
578. Seltzer CC, Bosse R, Garvey AJ. Mail survey response by smoking status. *Am J Epidemiol* 1974;100:453–7.

579. Seltzer CC, Jablon S. Effects of selection on mortality. *Am J Epidemiol* 1974;100:367–72.

580. Selwyn BJ, Frerichs RR, Smith GS, Olson J. Rapid epidemiologic assessment: the evolution of a new discipline. *Int J Epidemiol* 1989; 18(suppl 2):1.

581. Sempos CT, Johnson NE, Smith EL, Gilligan C. Effects of intra-individual and interindividual variation in repeated dietary records. *Am J Epidemiol* 1985;121:120–30.

582. Severson RK, Heuser L, Davis S. Recontacting study participants in epidemiologic research. *Am J Epidemiol* 1988;127:1318–20.

583. Shai D, Rosenwaike I. Errors in reporting education on the death certificate: some findings for older male decedents from New York State and Utah. *Am J Epidemiol* 1989;130:188–92.

584. Shaw GM, Gold EB. Methodological considerations in the study of parental occupational exposures and congenital malformations in offspring. *Scand J Work Environ Health* 1988;14:344–55.

585. Sheikh K, Mattingly S. Investigating non-response bias in mail surveys. *J Epidemiol Comm Health* 1981;35:293–6.

586. Sherwin R. Controlled trials of the diet-heart hypothesis: some comments on the experimental unit. *Am J Epidemiol* 1978;108:92–9.

587. Shuster JJ, Cook B. Hospital or population controls: a discussion. *J Chron Dis* 1983;36:315–6.

588. Siemiatycki J. Friendly control bias. *J Clin Epidemiol* 1989;42:687–8.

589. Siemiatycki J, Dewar R, Richardson L. Costs and statistical power associated with five methods of collecting occupation exposure information for population-based case-control studies. *Am J Epidemiol* 1989;130:1236–46.

590. Siemiatycki J, Thomas DC. Biological models and statistical interactions: an example from multistage carcinogenesis. *Int J Epidemiol* 1981;10:383–7.

591. Silber ALM, Horwitz RI. Detection bias and relation of benign breast disease to breast cancer. *Lancet* 1986;1:638–40.

592. Sirken MG, Rosenberg HM, Chevarley FM, Curtin LR. The quality of cause-of-death statistics. *Am J Pub Health* 1987;77:137–9.

593. Smith A. Comments on 'Popper's philosophy for epidemiologists' by Carol Buck. Comment two. *Int J Epidemiol* 1975;4:171–2.

594. Smith AH, Pearce NE, Callas PW. Cancer case-control studies with other cancers as controls. *Int J Epidemiol* 1988;17:298–306.

595. Smith GS. Development of rapid epidemiologic assessment methods to evaluate health status and delivery of health services. *Int J Epidemiol* 1989;18(suppl 2):2–15.

596. Smith J, Connett J, McHugh R. Planning the size of a matched case-control study for estimation of the odds ratio. *Am J Epidemiol* 1985;122:345–7.

597. Smith PG, Day NE. The design of case-control studies: the influence of confounding and interaction effects. *Int J Epidemiol* 1984;13:356–65.

598. Smith W. Randomization and optimal design. *J Chron Dis* 1983;36: 609–12.

599. Snow J. On the mode of communication of cholera (second edition). Churchill, London 1855.

600. Sobell J, Block G, Koslowe P et al. Validation of a retrospective questionnaire assessing diet 10-15 years ago. *Am J Epidemiol* 1989;130: 173–87.

601. Sosenko JM, Gardner LB. Attribute frequency and misclassification bias. *J Chron Dis* 1987;40:203–7.

602. Soskolne CL. Epidemiology: questions of science, ethics, morality, and law. *Am J Epidemiol* 1989;129:1–18.

603. Spirtas R, Steinberg M, Wands RC, Weisburger EK. Identification and classification of carcinogens: procedures of the chemical substances threshold limit value committee, ACGIH. *Am J Pub Health* 1986;76:1232–5.

604. Spiteri MA, Cook DG, Clarke SW. Reliability of eliciting physical signs in examination of the chest. *Lancet* 1988;1:873–5.

605. Spitzer WO. Ideas and words: two dimensions for debates on case controlling. *J Chron Dis* 1985;38:541–2.

606. Spry VM, Hovell MF, Sallis JG et al. Recruiting survey respondents to mailed surveys: controlled trials of incentives and prompts. *Am J Epidemiol* 1989;130:166–72.

607. Stamler J. Opportunities and pitfalls in international comparisons related to patterns, trends and determinants of CHD mortality. *Int J Epidemiol* 1989;18(suppl 1):3–18.

608. Stanton B, Clemens J, Aziz KMA et al. Comparability of results obtained by two-week home maintained diarrheal calendar with two-week diarrheal recall. *Int J Epidemiol* 1987:16:595–601.

609. Staquet M, Rozencweig M, Lee YJ, Muggia FM. Methodology for the assessment of new dichotomous diagnostic tests. *J Chron Dis* 1981; 34:599–610.

610. Stavraky KM, Clarke EA. Hospital or population controls? An unanswered question. *J Chron Dis* 1983;36:301–7.

611. Stehr-Green JK, Jason JM, Evatt BL. Potential effect of revising the CDC surveillance case definition for AIDS. *Lancet* 1988;1:520–1.

612. Stein REK, Gortmaker SL, Perrin EC et al. Severity of illness: concepts and measurements. *Lancet* 1987;2:1506–9.

613. Stellman SD. The case of the missing eights. An object lesson in data quality assurance. *Am J Epidemiol* 1989;129:857–60.

614. Stewart AL. The reliability and validity of self-reported weight and height. *J Chron Dis* 1982;35:295–309.

615. Stewart AW, Jackson RT, Ford MA, Beaglehole R. Underestimation of relative weight by use of self-reported height and weight. *Am J Epidemiol* 1987;125:122–6.

616. Stoller A. Methodological problems in mental illness epidemiology. *Int J Epidemiol* 1974;3:119–24.

617. Stolley PD, Tonascia JA, Sartwell PE et al. Agreement rates between oral contraceptive users and prescribers in relation to drug use histories. *Am J Epidemiol* 1978;107:226–35.

618. Storm HH. Completeness of cancer registration in Denmark 1943-1966 and efficacy of record linkage procedures. *Int J Epidemiol* 1988;17:44–9.

619. Straatman H, Verbeek ALM, Peeters PHM. Etiologic and prevented fraction in case-control studies of screening. *J Clin Epidemiol* 1988; 41:807–8.

620. Stratford JM. Methods of assessing gingival and periodontal disease: a review. *Int J Epidemiol* 1975;4:79–86.

621. Suchman EA. An appraisal with implications for theoretical development of some epidemiological work on heart disease. *Millbank Memorial Fund Quarterly* 1967;XIV(2):109–13.

622. Sun RK, Liff JM. Ascertainment bias of cervical carcinoma *in situ*. *Am J Pub Health* 1988;78:985.

623. Susser E, Susser M. Familial aggregation studies. A note on their epidemiologic properties. *Am J Epidemiol* 1989;129:23–30.

624. Susser M. Judgment and causal inference: criteria in epidemiologic studies. *Am J Epidemiol* 1977;105:1–15.

625. Susser M. The logic of Sir Karl Popper and the practice of epidemiology. *Am J Epidemiol* 1986;124:711–8. The author replies. *Am J Epidemiol* 1987;126:554–6.

626. Susser M. Epidemiology today: 'A thought-tormented world'. *Int J Epidemiol* 1989;18:481–8.

627. Swan SH, Petitti DB. A review of problems of bias and confounding in epidemiologic studies of cervical neoplasia and oral contraceptive use. *Am J Epidemiol* 1982;115:10–8.

628. Sweeney AM, Meyer MR, Aarons JH et al. Evaluation of methods for the prospective identification of early fetal losses in environmental epidemiology studies. *Am J Epidemiol* 1988;127:843–50.

629. Syme SL. Life style intervention in clinic-based trials. *Am J Epidemiol* 1978;108:87–91.

630. Taylor JW. Simple estimation of population attributable risk from case-control studies. *Am J Epidemiol* 1977;106:260.

631. Taylor R. Causation. Pp 56-66 in the Encyclopedia of Philosophy, vol II (ed: Edwards P) MacMillan, London 1967.

632. Terris M (ed). Goldberger on pellagra. Louisiana State University Press, Baton Rouge 1964.

633. Terris M. The changing relationships of epidemiology and society: the Robert Cruikshank lecture. J Public Health Policy. 1985;15–36.

634. Thomas DC, Greenland S. The relative efficiencies of matched and independent sample designs for case-control studies. *J Chron Dis* 1983;36:685–97.

635. Thompson FE, Lamphiear DE, Metzner HL et al. Reproducibility of reports of frequency of food use in the Tecumseh diet methodology study. *Am J Epidemiol* 1987;125:658–71.

636. Thompson WD. Statistical criteria in the interpretation of epidemiologic data. *Am J Pub Health* 1987a;77:191–4.

637. Thompson WD. On the comparison of effects. *Am J Pub Health* 1987b;77:491–2.

638. Thompson WD, Kelsey JL, Walter SD. Cost and efficiency in the

choice of matched and unmatched case-control study designs. *Am J Epidemiol* 1982;116:840–51.

639. Tilley BC, Barnes AB, Bergstralh E et al. A comparison of pregnancy history recall and medical records. Implications for retrospective studies. *Am J Epidemiol* 1985;121:269–81.

640. Tsai SP, Wen CP. The impact of competing risks on relative risk in occupational cohort studies. *Int J Epidemiol* 1984;13:518–25.

641. Tsai SP, Wen CP. A review of methodological issues of the standardized mortality ratio (SMR) in occupational cohort studies. *Int J Epidemiol* 1986;15:8–21.

642. Tunstall-Pedoe H. Diagnosis, measurement and surveillance of coronary events. *Int J Epidemiol* 1989;18(suppl 1):169–173.

643. Tyroler HA. Methods in international studies: definition, ascertainment, measurement, analysis: overview. *Int J Epidemiol* 1989; 18(suppl 1):164–5.

644. Törnberg SA, Jakobsson KFS, Eklund GA. Stability and validity of a single serum cholesterol measurement in a prospective cohort study. *Int J Epidemiol* 1988;17:797–803.

645. US Department of Health, Education and Welfare. Interview data on chronic conditions compared with information derived from medical records. *DHEW,* series 2, No 23, 1967.

646. US Department of Health, Education and Welfare. A summary of studies of interviewing methodology. *DHEW,* series 2, No 69, 1977.

647. van Beresteyn ECH, van't Hof MA, van der Heiden-Winkeldermaat HJ et al. Evaluation of the usefulness of the cross-check dietary history method in longitudinal studies. *J Chron Dis* 1987;40:1051–8.

648. Van den Brandt PA, Willett WC, Tannenbaum SR. Assessment of dietary nitrate intake by a self-administered questionnaire and by overnight urinary measurement. *Int J Epidemiol* 1989;18:852–7.

649. Vandenbroucke JP. Is the randomized controlled trial the real paradigm in epidemiology. *J Chron Dis* 1986;39:572.

650. Vandenbroucke JP. Should we abandon statistical modeling altogether. *Am J Epidemiol* 1987a;126:10–3.

651. Vandenbroucke JP. A short note on the history of the randomized controlled trial. *J Chron Dis* 1987b;40:985–7.

652. Vandenbroucke JP. Those who were wrong. *Am J Epidemiol* 1989; 130:3–5.

653. Vandenbroucke JP, Pardoel VPAM. An autopsy of epidemiologic methods: the case of "Poppers" in the early epidemic of the acquired immunodeficiency syndrome (AIDS). *Am J Epidemiol* 1989;129: 455–7.

654. Vandenbroucke JP, Vandenbroucke-Grauls CMJE. A note on the history of the calculation of hospital statistics. *Am J Epidemiol* 1988;127:699–702.

655. Van Leeuwen FE, de Vet HCW, Hayes RB et al. An assessment of the relative validity of retrospective interviewing for measuring dietary intake. *Am J Epidemiol* 1983;118:752–8.

656. van Staveren WA, Burema J, Deurenberg P, Katan MB. Weak associa-

tions in nutritional epidemiology: the importance of replication of observations on individuals. *Int J Epidemiol* 1988;17(suppl):964–9.

657. van Staveren WA, Deurenberg P, Katan MB et al. Validity of the fatty acid composition of subcutaneous fat tissue microbiopsies as an estimate of the long-term average fatty acid composition of the diet of separate individuals. *Am J Epidemiol* 1986;123:455–63.

658. van Staveren WA, West CE, Hoffmans MDAF et al. Comparison of contemporaneous and retrospective estimates of food consumption made by a dietary history method. *Am J Epidemiol* 1986;123:884–93.

659. Vessey MP. Some methodological problems in the investigation of rare adverse reactions to oral contraceptives. *Am J Epidemiol* 1971; 94:202–9.

660. Vinni K, Hakama M. Healthy worker effect in the total Finnish population. *Br J Ind Med* 1980;37:180–4.

661. Wacholder S, Boivin J-F. External comparisons with the case-cohort design. *Am J Epidemiol* 1987;126:1198–1209.

662. Walker AM. Proportion of disease attributable to the combined effect of two factors. *Int J Epidemiol* 1981;10:81–5.

663. Walker AM. Anamorphic analysis: sampling and estimation for covariate effects when both exposure and disease are known. *Biometrics* 1982;38:1025–32.

664. Walker AM. Misclassified confounders. *Am J Epidemiol* 1985;122: 921–2.

665. Walker AM. Reporting the results of epidemiologic studies. *Am J Pub Health* 1986a;76:556–8.

666. Walker AM. Significance tests represent consensus and standard practice. *Am J Pub Health* 1986b;76:1033. Erratum 1087.

667. Walker AM, Blettner M. Comparing imperfect measures of exposure. *Am J Epidemiol* 1985;121:783–90.

668. Walker AM, Martin-Moreno JM, Artalejo FR. Odd man out: a graphical approach to meta-analysis. *Am J Pub Health* 1988;78:961–6.

669. Walter SD. Berkson's bias and its control in epidemiologic studies. *J Chron Dis* 1980;33:721–5.

670. Walter SD. Effects of interaction, confounding and observational error on attributable risk estimation. *Am J Epidemiol* 1983;117: 598–604.

671. Walter SD. Assessment of the working lifetime risk of exposure in an occupational cohort. *Am J Epidemiol* 1989;129:230–1.

672. Walter SD, Clarke EA, Hatcher J, Stitt LW. A comparison of physician and patient reports of Pap smear histories. *J Clin Epidemiol* 1988; 41:401–10.

673. Walter SD, Holford TR. Additive, multiplicative, and other models for disease risks. *Am J Epidemiol* 1978;108:341–6.

674. Walter SD, Irwig LM. Estimation of test error rates, disease prevalence and relative risk from misclassified data: a review. *J Clin Epidemiol* 1988;41:923–37.

675. Walter SD, Marrett LD, Mishkel N. Effect of contact letter on control response rates in cancer studies. *Am J Epidemiol* 1988;127:691–4.

676. Wang J-D, Miettinen OS. Occupational mortality studies. Principles of validity. *Scand J Work Environ Health* 1982;8:153–8.
677. Warner SC, Aldrich TE. The status of cancer cluster investigations undertaken by state health departments. *Am J Pub Health* 1988; 78:306–7.
678. Washburn RA, Montoye HJ. The assessment of physical activity by questionnaire. *Am J Epidemiol* 1986;123:563–76.
679. Waters WE. Ethics and epidemiological research. *Int J Epidemiol* 1985;14:48–51.
680. Watkins CJ, Burton P, Leeder S et al. Doctor diagnosis and maternal recall of lower respiratory illness. *Int J Epidemiol* 1982;11:62–6.
681. Weddell JM. Registers and registries: a review. *Int J Epidemiol* 1973;2:221–8.
682. Weed DL. On the logic of causal inference. *Am J Epidemiol* 1986; 123:965–79. The author replies. *Am J Epidemiol* 1987a;126: 157–8. The author replies. *Am J Epidemiol* 1987b;126:557.
683. Weed DL, Selmon M, Sinks T. Links between categories of interaction. *Am J Epidemiol* 1988;127:17–27.
684. Weeks MF, Kulka RA, Lessler JT, Whitmore RW. Personal versus telephone surveys for collecting household health data at the local level. *Am J Pub Health* 1983;73:1389–94.
685. Weiss NS. Inferring causal relationships. Elaboration of the criterion of "dose-response". *Am J Epidemiol* 1981;113:487–90.
686. Weiss NS. Measuring the separate effects of low parity and its antecedents on the incidence of ovarian cancer. *Am J Epidemiol* 1988; 128:451–5.
687. Weiss NS, Daling JR, Chow WH. Control definition in case-control studies of ectopic pregnancy. *Am J Pub Health* 1985;75:67–8.
688. Wells CK, Feinstein AR. Detection bias in the diagnostic pursuit of lung cancer. *Am J Epidemiol* 1988;128:1016–26.
689. Werler MM, Pober BR, Nelson K, Holmes LB. Reporting accuracy among mothers of malformed and nonmalformed infants. *Am J Epidemiol* 1989;129:415–21.
690. West DW, Schuman KL, Lyon JL et al. Differences in risk estimations from a hospital and a population-based case-control study. *Int J Epidemiol* 1984;13:235–9.
691. White E. The effect of misclassification of disease status in follow-up studies: implications for selecting disease classification criteria. *Am J Epidemiol* 1986;124:816–25.
692. White E. Re: Exposure opportunity in epidemiologic studies. *Am J Epidemiol* 1988;128:245.
693. Wiener Z, Abelson A, Herman J. The diagnostic process—some unwitting uses. *J Clin Epidemiol* 1989;42:377–9.
694. Wiklund K, Einhorn J, Wennström G, Rapaport E. A Swedish cancer environment register available for research. *Scand J Work Environ Health* 1981;7:64–7.
695. Wilcox AJ, Russell IT. Perinatal mortality: standardizing for birthweight is biased. *Am J Epidemiol* 1983;118:857–64.

696. Willett W. Nutritional epidemiology: issues and challenges. *Int J Epidemiol* 1987;16(suppl):312–7.
697. Willett WC, Sampson L, Browne ML et al. The use of a self-administered questionnaire to assess diet four years in the past. *Am J Epidemiol* 1988;127:188–99.
698. Willett WC, Sampson L, Stampfer MJ et al. Reproducibility and validity of a semiquantitative food frequency questionnaire. *Am J Epidemiol* 1985;122:51–65.
699. Willett W, Stampfer MJ. Total energy intake: implications for epidemiologic analyses. *Am J Epidemiol* 1986;124:17–27.
700. Williams OD. Methodological issues in international comparisons. *Int J Epidemiol* 1989;18(suppl 1): 166–8.
701. Wingo PA, Ory HW, Layde PM et al. The evaluation of the data collection process for a multicenter, population-based, case-control design. *Am J Epidemiol* 1988;128:206–17.
702. Wong O. Further criticisms on epidemiological methodology in occupational studies. *J Occup Med* 1977;19:220–2.
703. Wu ML, Whittemore AS, Jung DL. Errors in reported dietary intakes. I. Short-term recall. *Am J Epidemiol* 1986;124:826–35.
704. Wu ML, Whittemore AS, Jung DL. Errors in reported dietary intakes. II. Long-term recall. *Am J Epidemiol* 1988;128:1137–45.
705. Zelen M. A new design for randomized clinical trials. *N Engl J Med* 1979;300:1242–5.
706. Zelen M. Commentary on "Randomization and optimal design". *J Chron Dis* 1983;36:613–4.

Subject Index

A

Accuracy, 4,113
Age
   as confounder, 23,27
   incidence rate effects,
      39,40
   misclassification effects,
      31
Aggregated data, 96–97
Association, 1–3
   causal, 104–106
   confounders and, 21–22,
      101,102
   of exposure/disease
      onset, 93
   of exposure/disease
      prevalence, 93–94
   generalizibility, 106–107
   interpretation, 101–107
   misclassification effects,
      28–30,42,101–102
   power of, 111–112
   random error and, 101,
      102
   statistical, 103–105

B

Bias. *See* Systematic error,
      selection bias
Body mass index, 82,137

C

Case, definition, 113
Case-control study, 5,6,
      55–60,97

   choice of, 87–90
   cohort study versus,
      87–90
   cumulative incidence, 57
   definition, 55,113
   design(s), 57–58
   design type A, 61–64,88
      efficiency, 63–64,67,89
      exposure, 97
      follow-up, 62
      selection of controls,
         61,62
      systematic errors,
         62–63,98
   design type B, 65–69,88
      efficiency, 67,68–69,89
      exposure, 66–68 97
      follow-up, 65–66,68
      misclassification,
         67–68
      nonparticipation, 68,
         102
      selection of controls,
         65,89
      study base, 65
      study population, 65
      systematic errors,
         66–67,98
      validity, 66–68
   design type C, 71–75,88
      efficiency, 74–75,89
      exposure, 71,72–74,97
      nonparticipation, 102
      selection of controls,
         71–74,89
      study base, 71,74
      systematic errors,

Case-control study (*contd.*)
72–74,98,
102–103
efficiency, 43,63–64,87,
88
cohort study compari-
son, 55,59,60
exposure frequency, 88
follow-up, 62
incidence, 89–90
incidence rate, 56–57
induction time, 90
interpretation of results,
102–103
matched, 99
nested, 99
power of association,
111–112
principles of, 55–56
relative risk, 55–56
selection of controls,
33,34,56–58,61,62
case matching, 58–59
number of, 59,60
as random sample, 57
study base, 55
subdivisions, 97–99
systematic errors,
59–60,62–63
Causality, 104–106
Chimney sweeps, 25–26,
29–30
Cohort study, 6,97
case-control versus,
87–90
choice of, 87–90
of closed population, 5–6

cost of, 38–39
definition, 7,113
disease diagnosis, 16–17
efficiency, 6,55,59,60,
87–88
examination of exposure
conditions, 41
exposure, 12–15,27,39,
88,98
incidence, 89
induction time, 88
power of association, 111
precision, 6
principles of, 8–17,55,56
retrospective, 99
stages, 10
study base, 8,10–11
study population, 12–15
systematic errors, 98
Confidence interval,
36–37,101
Confounders
age as, 23,27
association and, 21–22,
101,102
in case-control study, 74
definition, 1,20,113
disease development
effects, 21
empirical, 2
exposure and, 22,24–27
lack of information
regarding, 42
relative risk and, 22
as risk indicator, 21–22
study design choice and,
88

systematic errors and,
22–23
theoretical, 2
unknown, 90–91,92
validity, 88
Confounding
control of, 104
data analysis-related, 34
definition, 1,20,114
systematic errors and,
20–27
Controls
case matching,
58–59,114–115
deceased, 73
definition, 55
hospital, 71–73
number of, 59,60
selection of, 56–58,65,89
in case-control type A
study, 61,62
in case-control study
type B, 65,89
in case-control study
type C, 71–74,89
neighbor controls,
73–74
as random sample, 57
as systematic error
source, 103
Cost-efficiency. *See*
Efficiency
Covariance, 20–21,104
of aggregated data, 96–97
of risk indicators, 23–24
Cross-sectional study,
93–96

exposure misclassifica-
tion, 94
study population, 95

D
Data, epidemiologic
aggregated, 96–97
register of, 11,41–43
storage, 61–63
unprocessed, 61–62
"Diluting effect", 19
Disease
diagnosis, cost of, 89
occurrence follow-up,
16–17,42–43
risk indicators, 22,
23–24,116
Dose-response pattern,
104–105,114
Double-blind study, 92

E
Effect modification, 3,114
Efficiency, 5,38–43
of case-control study, 43,
87,88
cohort study compari-
son, 55,59,60
design type A, 63–64,
67,89
design type B, 67,
68–69,89
design type C, 74–75,
89
of cohort study, 6,87–88

Efficiency (*contd.*)
  case-control study
    comparison, 55,
      59,60
  definition, 35,38,113
  exposure frequency and,
    39,40
  factors affecting, 11,
    38–43
  disease occurrence
    follow-up, 42–43
  exposure conditions
    examination,
    41–42
  study base, 39–41
  improvement, 35
  of randomized study, 91
Epidemiologic investigation
  associations, 1–3
  subdivisions, 97–99
Epidemiology
  definition, 1,114
  terminology of, 1–6
Errors
  confounding. *See*
    Confounders
  random. *See* Random
    error
  systematic. *See*
    Systematic error
Examination methods,
  14–15
  blunted, 28
Experiment, definition, 114
Experimental study, 90–93
Exposure, 1–2
  biological effects, 105

in case-control study, 71,
  72–74,88
design type A, 97
design type B, 66–68,
  97
design type C, 71,
  72–74,97
in cohort study, 12,27,
  88,98
confounding factors, 22,
  24–27
cost of information,
  88–89
definition, 12–13,114
effect modification, 3
efficiency and, 39,40
examination of
  conditions, 41–42
frequency, 88
individuals' health status
  and, 24
induction period, 13–14
intervention study, 90–91
level of, 15
lifestyle and, 24–26
misclassification,
  6,27–30,33,88,
  106–107
association and,
  101–102
in cross-sectional
  study, 94
study design choice
  and, 88
multiple, 2,72
precision and, 15
random assignment, 7

study base size and, 38
subdivisions, 47–48,
121–122

F
False negative findings, 103
False positive findings, 103
Follow-up, 42–43
in case-control study,
62,65–66,68
definition, 4,114
Follow-up study. *See*
Cohort study

G
Gender, as confounder, 23
Generalizability, 114

H
Healthy worker effect, 24
Henle-Koch postulates, 104

I
Incidence
of case-control study,
57,89–90
of cohort study, 89
cumulative, 9–10,57,114
definition, 1,93,114
of prevalence study,
93–96
study base size and, 38
study design choice and,
87–88

Incidence rate, 9
age factors, 39,40
of case-control study,
56–57
definition, 114
Induction time, 13–14,88
of case-control study, 90
of cohort study, 13–14,88
definition, 2,114
variability, 13
Interpretation, of results,
101–107
causality and, 104–106
generalizability and,
106–107
Intervention study, 90–93,
99

L
Latent period, 114
Lifestyle, exposure and,
24–26

M
Matching, of case controls,
58–59,114–115
overmatching, 58
of unexposed to
exposed, 115
Misclassification
association and, 101–102
definition, 115
disease-related, 27,
30–32,88
association and, 102

Misclassification (*contd.*)
   study design choice
      and, 88
   exposure-related,
      6,27–30,33,88,
      106–107
   association and,
      101–102
   of cross-sectional
      study, 94
   study design choice
      and, 88
Misclassification,
      nondifferential
   of case-control study,
      67–68
   data register and, 42
   definition, 115
   negative findings and,
      103
Mortality, standardized
   ratio, 116

N
Negative findings, 103
Nonparticipation, 33,68,
      102
   case control matching
      and, 58–59

O
Occupational factors,
      exposure and,
      24–26
Overmatching, 58

P
Penetration, power of,
      91–92
Person-time, 115
Population. *See also* Study
      population
   definition, 115
   register of, 66
Power
   of association, 111–112
   calculations, 37–38
   of penetration, 91–92
Precision
   of cohort study, 6
   definition, 5,35,115
   exposure level
      correlation, 15
   negative findings and,
      103
   random error and, 35–38
Prevalence, 1
Prevalence study. *See*
      Cross-sectional study

R
Random error, 5,35–43,
      101,106. *See also*
      Efficiency
   association and, 101,102
   in cohort study, 14
   definition, 35,115
   precision and, 35–38
   adequacy, 37
   improvement, 36
Randomized experiment,
      90–93,99

limitations of, 7
Random sample, of study
  base, 74,98
Random variation, 35–36
Rate ratio. *See* Relative risk
Register
  of disease, 66
  of epidemiologic data,
    11,41–42
  follow-up and, 42–43
  of population, 66
Relative risk
  2%, 110
  10%, 109–110
  50%, 109
  of case-control study,
    55–56
  confidence intervals,
    36,101
  confounders and, 22
  of cross-sectional study,
    94
  definition, 9,115–116
  misclassification effects,
    30,31–32
  systematic errors and, 19
Reproducibility. *See*
    Precision
Research grant
    applications, 37
Risk factor, 116
Risk indicator, 22,23–24,
    116

S
Sensitivity

definition, 116
of disease classification,
    31
of exposure, 28
statistical calculation,
    109–110
Specificity
  definition, 116
  of disease classification,
    31
  of exposure, 28
  statistical calculation,
    109–110
Specimens, storage of,
    61–62
Standardized mortality
    ratio, 116
Stratification, 116
Stratified analysis, 117
Stratified sampling, 117
Study base. *See also* Study
    population
  of case-control study,
    55,65,71,74
  choice of, 10–11
  of cohort study, 8,10–11
  definition, 4,5,117
  efficiency and, 39–41
  exposure frequency, 40
  generalizibility of results
    and, 106–107
  misclassification, 32
  precision and, 38–41
  as random sample, 74,98
  size, 11,36–37,38
Study design. *See also*
    Case-control study;

Study design (*contd.*)
    Cohort study;
    Cross-sectional
    study; Ecologic
    study; Experimental
    study
    definition, 4–6
    factors affecting, 87–99
      cohort versus
        case-control
        designs, 87–90
      confounders, 88
      diagnosis cost, 89
      disease incidence,
        87–88
      exposure information,
        88
      exposure information
        cost, 88–89
      induction period, 88
      misclassification, 88
      possibility of
        abstention, 89
      selection of controls, 89
Study population
    of case-control study, 65
    closed, 3–4,8,99,113
    of cohort study, 8,12–15
    of cross-sectional study,
      95
    definition, 3–4,33–34,
      113
    of nested case-control
      study, 99
    open, 4,114
    random sample, 80,133,

      134–135
    selection bias, 33–34
Systematic error,
    4–5,19–34,20–27,
    106. *See also*
    Confounders
    of case-control study,
      59–60
      design type A, 62–63,
        98
      design type B, 66–67,
        98
      design type C, 72–74,
        98,102–103
    of cohort study, 6,98
    confounding/con-
      founders, 20–27
    definition, 19,117
    misclassification, 27–33
    of prevalence study,
      93–96
    selection bias, 33–34,
      94–95
    sources of, 101
    study population-related,
      33–34
    subdivision, 34

V
Validity
    of case-control study,
      66–68
    of confounders, 8819,117
    definition, 4–5,19,117